The 7-Day Allergy Makeover

"Allergies can manifest in everything, from the food you eat to what you keep in your bedroom closet. In her new book *The 7-Day Allergy Makeover*, Dr. Bennett shows you obvious and not-so-obvious allergen sources and provides concrete steps to eliminate those allergies. Highly recommended!"

> —JJ Virgin, CNS, CHFS, host and costar of TLC's *Freaky Eaters* and author of the *New York Times* bestseller *The Virgin Diet*

"Dr. Bennett has developed a foolproof method for reversing the serious problems encountered when someone suffers from allergies. I highly recommend her book and think it will change the lives of those that use it."

> —Marcelle Pick, RNC, MSN, OB/GYN NP, cofounder of Women to Women and author of *Are You Tired and Wired?* and *The Core Balance Diet*

"If allergy symptoms have taken over your life or your child's life, you simply cannot afford to be without Dr. Bennett's groundbreaking program."

> —Dr. Todd LePine, MD, physician at Dr. Mark Hyman's Ultra Wellness Center and clinical medical director of Metametrix Laboratories

"*The 7-Day Allergy Makeover* is the first book that gives people the ability to control their own allergies. Dr. Susanne Bennett has done a phenomenal job making this complex topic simple and laying out the easy steps that will reverse years of symptoms."

> —Alan Christianson, NMD, author of *The Complete Idiot's Guide to Thyroid Disease*

"*The 7-Day Allergy Makeover* is an easy-to-follow and complete road map to a healthier and allergy-free you. The quality of your life in all aspects is about to change once you read her book."

> —Dr. Charles Sophy, DO, celebrity psychiatrist and author of *Side by Side: The Revolutionary Mother-Daughter Program for Conflict-Free Communication*

continued . . .

"If you have children, you should not miss *The 7-Day Allergy Makeover*. Children's allergies don't just come from food, but also toys, pets, and hundreds of common household products. Dr. Bennett will guide you through this maze to better health for you and your family."

—Steven Masley, MD, FAAFP, CNS, FACN, author of
The 30 Day Heart Tune-Up and *Ten Years Younger*

"I have been a patient of Dr. Susanne Bennett for eight years. I am very grateful to her and see the results of all her work continuing to blossom in my life."

—Hallie Foote, award-winning Broadway and film actor

"Allergies are the key to many symptoms and conditions—ones that you may never even associate with an allergy! Dr. Susanne Bennett will help you uncover the underlying causes of your hard-to-treat, difficult and even disabling conditions, so you can remove the cause and move forward to enjoy full, vibrant health. This book holds the key: read it and live life as well as it can be!"

—Hyla Cass, MD, author of *Eight Weeks to Vibrant Health*

"Dr. Susanne Bennett is one of the handful of health professionals I personally turn to when I want advice for myself or my family. Even if you don't have allergies, you should read this book. It's a treasure trove of information about how exposures to common foods and substances can influence your health. *The 7-Day Allergy Makeover* is a must-read for everyone!"

—Jonny Bowden, PhD, CNS, author of *The 150 Healthiest Foods on Earth*
and *The Great Cholesterol Myth*

"Dr. Susanne Bennett's *7-Day Allergy Makeover* is a clear and powerful system by a seasoned and experienced expert. You will not only feel better in seven days, but you will be on the road to lifelong health after reading this book."

—Dr. Nalini Chilkov, founder of Integrative Cancer Answers

"My family and I have been patients of Dr. Susanne Bennett for over seven years. If you follow her advice, diet, and recommendations you will feel so much clearer, healthier, and vibrant. Highly recommended!"

—Lavinia Errico, founder of Equinox

THE
7-Day Allergy
Makeover

A Simple Program to
Eliminate Allergies and
Restore Vibrant Health
from the Inside Out

Dr. Susanne Bennett

A PERIGEE BOOK

A PERIGEE BOOK
Published by the Penguin Group
Penguin Group (USA) LLC
375 Hudson Street, New York, New York 10014

USA • Canada • UK • Ireland • Australia • New Zealand • India • South Africa • China

penguin.com

A Penguin Random House Company

Library of Congress Cataloging-in-Publication Data

Bennett, Susanne, 1962–
The 7-day allergy makeover : a simple program to eliminate allergies
and restore vibrant health from the inside out / Dr. Susanne Bennett.
pages   cm
"A Perigee Book."
Includes bibliographical references and index.
ISBN 978-0-399-16624-2
1. Allergy.   2. Allergy—Treatment.   3. Allergens—Control—Environmental aspects.
I. Title.   II. Title: Seven-day allergy makeover.
RC584.B43   2014
616.97—dc23   2013039971

First edition: March 2014

PRINTED IN THE UNITED STATES OF AMERICA

10   9   8   7   6   5   4   3   2   1

Text design by Tiffany Estreicher

Most Perigee books are available at special quantity discounts for bulk purchases for sales
promotions, premiums, fund-raising, or educational use. Special books, or book excerpts, can also
be created to fit specific needs. For details, write: Special.Markets@us.penguingroup.com.

CONTENTS

INTRODUCTION

....

....

CODY'S STORY

....

If not for that fateful Valentine's Day some twenty years ago, I never would have become an allergist. I never would have discovered how to heal allergies naturally and permanently. And you wouldn't have this book in your hands!

Cody was truly a love child, conceived on the very day we dedicate to love: February 14. My pregnancy was amazingly easy—I was high on pregnancy hormones and, at thirty-one years old, at my healthiest and most vibrant. I exercised regularly, ate all the "right" foods: nondairy and gluten free (before anyone even talked much about gluten), organic veggies, vitamins, and fish oils. I drank only purified water, avoided sodas and alcohol. I gained only eighteen pounds, and almost ten of those were Cody—well, nine pounds and eleven ounces, to be precise.

Then I went into labor, and that's when things got rough. Because of my small frame, after thirty hours in the hospital, I had to have a cesarean section. Even with all the painkillers and epidural drugs pumped into me, I will never forget the way my son appeared when the doctor pulled him out of my belly. Cody was *huge*—more like a three-month-old than a newborn. Newborns are usually "floppy," without any muscle tone in the neck, but my minutes-old son was turning his head left and right, checking out the room. I honestly believe he was looking for me! My doctor put Cody on my breast, and he latched right on.

I understood at that moment that my purpose in life was to be his protector and life source. And I would need to be all that—more than I could ever have imagined.

We brought him home, and the first couple of months, George and I had the marvelous, glorious experience of living with a newborn. Cody was truly the love of my life. Until then, I never knew I could feel that much joy.

But that idyllic state was not to last. The love and joy continued, but before I knew it my joyous existence was pervaded with worry. Anxiety. Sadness. Despair. And even fear for Cody's life.

At just three months old, Cody became plagued by allergies. I don't mean a simple sneezing fit or a rash that subsided in a few days. Without explanation, he began to show a whole range of severe allergic reactions, including hives; loose, mucus-filled stool; a constantly runny nose; intense rashes; and respiratory distress (wheezing) during viral infections. His pediatrician thought nothing of it—said it was typical for newborn babies. I left feeling somewhat consoled, but given the severity of Cody's suffering, my suspicions lingered.

Then the turning point came. At six months old, Cody had an eczema rash under his chin that simply would not go away. We even used a strong cortisone cream given to us by his pediatrician. Being a doctor myself, I knew something wasn't clicking, and I started looking for deeper reasons why he was so sensitive and reactive. I decided to approach the issue as any scientist would: by conducting a controlled experiment. I shaved off his newborn hair and sent it into a reputable laboratory. What they found was astounding: high levels of nickel and mercury—in his *hair*!

Where would a baby be picking up these toxic metals? I dived into research. I went to my favorite medical library at the University of California at Los Angeles (UCLA), scoured the Internet, and read everything I could find on these chemicals. Before long, I found out that nickel is a known common cause of skin rashes and allergic reactions. A first clue! I remembered experiencing something similar when I was a teenager. Every time I wore costume jewelry—jewelry not made of real gold—I would develop a rash on my earlobes until I stopped wearing it. "Nickel allergy—like mother, like son!" I thought.

My mind was racing. Where was Cody being exposed to nickel? All his meals were made of organic pureed food. But then it hit me: every time we fed him we were using *stainless-steel* spoons. Not only that but all our pots and pans were made of stainless steel or aluminum. I quickly replaced all our cookware with iron, glass, and enamel, which tend to be nonallergenic. I started using wooden and porcelain spoons for Cody's meals, and—surprise, surprise!—within a week, the rash under his chin went away.

I was elated. I thought that with a little scientific knowledge, detective work, and homegrown experimentation, I had cured his allergies. Wishful thinking! Although the rash under the chin did subside, we had only begun what was to become a three-year battle with allergy symptoms. From this time until his first birthday, Cody started to experience other allergies: constant nasal congestion and runny nose, frequent colds, hives, and rashes on the face and body. He had several respiratory distress illnesses that the doctors finally diagnosed as asthma, which, as you may know, is a breathing condition in which the respiratory airways constrict, making breathing difficult. Eczema and rhinitis (inflammation of the mucous membranes in the nasal passages) were a daily thing, but this time around, the doctors couldn't really help. The drugs they prescribed for rhinitis made his heart race and made him anxious and nervous. The cortisone creams worked only half the time. That left the other half. And when his entire body was red and inflamed, it was impossible to cover it all with the cream. I knew that too much cortisone could be harmful for a child's delicate skin and body. I grew despondent, troubled. I turned to George, my family, and friends for support, but it seemed as if things would never improve.

Then an idea struck me: Cody's hair analysis had said he had high levels of not just nickel but also mercury. It was time to hit the research trail once again. After a time, I learned about a condition called *fetal metal syndrome.* Children with this syndrome absorbed the heavy metals the mother was exposed to while they were in the womb. So I racked my brain: when was I exposed to mercury? In the early 1990s, not one doctor or pregnancy book recommended that pregnant women refrain from eating fish and other seafoods. The breaking news about tuna possibly being dangerous for pregnancy and fetal development came out years later. Without knowing the consequences of what I was doing, I had eaten tuna three or four times a week during my pregnancy. Mercury had made its way into Cody in utero. That was the second clue.

But the mercury mystery had another twist. I went to my dentist and found out that I had three amalgam fillings (silver to gray in color, depending on the age of the filling), and one, which was made of a mercury alloy (mercury, silver, tin, zinc, and copper) had a large crack in it. My dentist said that most likely the filling was leaching out mercury the entire time I was pregnant and nursing. I was swallowing minute amounts of mercury every time I chewed hard food! Not only that, but every time I drank liquids over 105°F, the toxic heavy metal would vaporize, and I could contaminate myself by breathing it in.

The terrible truth: I was poisoning my baby with my own breast milk. That night, I cried even harder than all those other nights when I just couldn't understand what was hurting Cody. Now I understood, and it was monstrously hard to accept. *I* was hurting Cody. And maybe I was too late. Intuitively, Cody never wanted to nurse from my right breast—the same side where my cracked amalgam filling was located (lower right jaw). I had to pump the right side to keep the breast from drying up. But I had nursed him with toxic breast milk for a *full year* before he weaned himself off it on his own. The guilt was staggering.

To this day, I have yet to find a child or adult with the high levels of mercury my son had at six months old. How do you deal with a child who reacts to so many foods that it seems almost impossible to feed him? Eggs, strawberries, *all* nuts, bananas, most vegetables—all these were off the list of foods he could eat. At the worst point, Cody could eat, literally, only ten foods without suffering an allergic reaction—usually a rash or breathing difficulties, or both. And what do you do if that same child begins coughing and wheezing just from entering a room filled with perfume, air fresheners, or the scent of rubber? And what can you do if medical interventions only make everything worse? That was the terrifying situation I faced with my son every day of his early life.

For the first two years, I took Cody to a variety of doctors, trying to pinpoint the cause of his distress and illness. They just put him on a lot of drugs. And I mean a *lot*. In spite of the drugs, he still had to be rushed to the emergency room several times for anaphylactic reactions to strawberries, molds, dairy, and latex. One time, he had serious trouble breathing because we went into a sporting-goods store that had lots of rubber-soled shoes. The smell triggered a reaction (latex allergy) that constricted his breathing. Another time, he ate a small bite of an apple pie from the local grocery store and his throat closed up rapidly during his sleep. I sent a sample of the apple pie to be analyzed by a lab, and they found that it was contaminated with *Penicillium* mold! So all those foods, rubber, mold—and there was more to come.

Things got so bad, my doctor advised us to carry an EpiPen— an emergency medical injection that would immediately give the proper dose of epinephrine to open up his airway, eliminating ana-phylactic symptoms, and save his life. The thought of having to use the EpiPen was scary for us. I became the mother of all helicopter mothers, hovering over my child because he was constantly react-ing to *everything*. This wasn't what I wanted for myself, but more important, it wasn't what I wanted for him.

When Cody was just about a year and a half old he had a rou-tine vaccine injection for chicken pox and MMR (measles, mumps, and rubella). The vaccination caused a raging 106°F fever, and within days, Cody couldn't walk without falling over. He looked as though he had muscle strength in his legs, but something else was faltering. I had no idea what was wrong, but I knew this shouldn't be happening. I immediately sought out medical advice. Both his pediatrician and two other doctors said that the vaccines couldn't be causing the loss of balance and lower-extremity motor skills. I didn't believe it. He had been fine and able to walk and run before getting vaccinated. Now he was wobbling and falling over.

Finally, a fourth doctor confirmed something very different from the first three: Cody had gotten cerebellar meningitis from the four vaccines (chicken pox, measles, mumps, and rubella). Clue three. His cerebellum was inflamed and irritated from the live attenuated viruses he had been injected with. The cerebellum is responsible for many different neurological functions, particularly balance and coordination of the body and extremities. I was scared beyond belief. Would Cody walk again? The doctor was hopeful that Cody's coordination would slowly come back so he could walk without falling over. Sure enough, within three weeks, he could do just that. But it wasn't easy going. Sometimes, he would trip over his own feet and fall flat on his belly. He became very clumsy, bumping into things other children wouldn't, and his hand-eye coordination was impaired. Being a toddler, he probably thought nothing of the side effects, but for a mother with medical knowledge, it was a bitter pill. Still, I felt that these side effects were minor issues compared to his inability to walk. I was just happy that he was back on his two feet, walking and running.

This nerve-racking experience was the straw that broke the camel's back. It was time for a real, permanent change.

FROM CONCERNED MOM TO ALLERGY SPECIALIST

At the time of Cody's severe allergy symptoms, I had a thriving sports medicine practice. Because I worked with physicians all the time, I could see the value of mainstream allopathic medicine for many situations, but clearly, my son's deteriorating condition was not one of them. After the cerebellar meningitis incident, I decided that it was up to *me* to be my son's doctor and healer. That decision was the beginning of getting Cody back on track. That was the start of the book you now hold in your hands.

I started reading more, researching more. I began piecing together all the clues about Cody's condition, from the heavy-metal allergies to food allergies, to his susceptibility to latex and chemical smells. At first, not all the pieces fit, but I knew I was onto something—a discovery of immense proportions.

As I mentioned earlier, I barely slept because I would go and check on Cody three or four times a night to make sure he was breathing freely. Nighttime was the best time for me to study because I had a full-time practice during the day. I was so driven to find *any* knowledge that could help my son, I seemed to have forgotten about almost everything else. It felt as if we were dealing with a ticking time bomb that I had to defuse. It terrified me, as it would any mother. I lived in constant dread.

As I write this paragraph, Cody is eighteen years old. He is completely free of all anaphylactic reactions and lives a happy, healthy life. What I was able to discover over the next few years about his allergies saved him from a life of suffering. It may even have saved his life.

Once I made the decision to become Cody's healer I read every book on allergies and environmental medicine I could get my hands on. In the spring of 1996, I begged the American Academy of Environmental Medicine (AAEM) to let me take its postgraduate courses, which are intended for doctors who hope to specialize in the science of allergies and environmental medicine. I really mean *begged* because only medical doctors were allowed to take their courses. I was a licensed chiropractic physician who would have no problem with understanding the concepts, terms, and methodologies of the courses. After many calls, many rejections, they finally said yes. I would be able to go through the postgraduate curriculum, but I was not allowed to participate in any of the medical practice techniques that were being taught. During these courses, I learned volumes of priceless wisdom from Dr. Doris Rapp, the queen of pediatric allergy medicine. Over countless sleepless nights, I came to understand allergies in a holistic way. First, I made Cody's *nutrition* his medicine and restored his intestinal terrain, his gut flora. I saw that it wasn't enough to keep him *away* from allergens; rather, I had to take proactive steps to increase his body's innate ability to deal with the molds, toxins, metals, and chemicals that are an inescapable part of our environment.

I changed my own practice from sports medicine to helping people who suffer from the sort of debilitating allergies that Cody had gone through. I took a whole battery of postgraduate courses and earned certifications in desensitization techniques, all relating to allergies: nutrition, environmental medicine, neuroimmunology, bioenergetic medicine, and even psychological medicine. At home, I cleaned up Cody's diet and our living environment in exactly the same way that this book will teach you to do. Desensitization techniques and nutritional supplementation using probiotics, digestive enzymes, vitamins, and minerals were also immensely helpful. By the time he was four years old, Cody was totally free of allergic reactions.

What began as a mother's desperate fight to save her son evolved into a comprehensive program that helps a broad range of allergy sufferers heal themselves naturally. Today I am a full-time natural allergy specialist. So far, I have logged in more than ninety thousand allergy patient visits, and I see roughly a hundred patients a week, ranging from children to working moms, from auto mechanics to movie stars. Most of them come to me after exhausting every possible resource: doctors, medicines, creams, shots—all the things that were used on Cody before I discovered the natural healing methods that *do* work. My patients suffer from hives, sneezing, headaches, asthma, muscle and joint pain, bloating and digestive problems, anaphylactic response symptoms, and much more. Today, their lives are transformed, and all without costly doctor visits, drugs, or surgery. The truth is, after watching Cody's suffering, after helping him heal, I know I can help *them* heal, too. What I have learned is more powerful than the worst allergy symptoms.

Simply put, *The 7-Day Allergy Makeover* condenses twenty-four years of clinical experience into an easy-to-implement plan for eliminating allergy symptoms from your life forever. In reading this book, you are making a choice to begin your life anew by letting your body heal itself from within.

This book could not be more timely. Allergic diseases affect as many as fifty million people in this country, and a nationwide survey found that more than half (54.6 percent) of all Americans test positive to one or more allergens. Mild allergy symptoms can make the sufferer feel fatigued, congested, and bloated, with a lack of motivation or an inability to concentrate. With severe allergy symptoms, individuals of any age can have such aggressive inflammatory reactions that they must use an EpiPen or go to the hospital. The cost of treating allergies in the United States alone is in the billions of dollars, placing a crushing demand on an already overburdened healthcare system.

But there is a bigger cost. What price tag can a parent place on an allergic child's comfort or their very life? How can we treat allergies to reduce lifelong disability and dependence on medications, shots, and breathing treatments?

> More than half (54.6 percent) of all Americans test positive to one or more allergens.

Like many doctors across all fields of medicine, I believe that a huge part of the allergy solution is *prevention*. But this is easier said than done, especially if you aren't even sure what is causing your reactions or making them worse. Each chapter in *The 7-Day Allergy Makeover* focuses on a different aspect of your health and environment. You will discover how lifestyle, diet, water, and even the layout of your home and workplace can cause allergies.

What if I told you the best way to fight pollen allergies might be to stop eating cheese? Or to drink cleaner water? Or to get dust mite covers for your pillows?

You see, allergies are not always simple and clear-cut. Sometimes the root issue is not necessarily the pollen itself, but a buildup of several different causes—a broader sensitivity that makes your body's immune system constantly reactive. Getting to the root of a pollen allergy means restoring your whole body to a healthier state. Reducing your immune reactivity will reduce your allergic reactions to pollen. And that's why we start the allergy makeover with food and water. Over so many years of clinical practice, I found that the easiest and *fastest* way to reduce your immune hypersensitivity is through *controlling what goes into your digestive system.* The more optimally you choose what to eat and drink, the better you can deal with pollen!

Once you understand what goes into creating allergies, you can modify certain aspects of your nutrition, air quality, living environment, body hygiene, and emotional stresses to create an allergy-free lifestyle.

IS THE 7-DAY ALLERGY MAKEOVER FOR ME?

First, *The 7-Day Allergy Makeover* is written for people who want to take an *active* role in their own healing. In contrast to the approach of conventional medicine, which often treats the *symptoms* and not the *causes*, healing your allergies naturally requires *your participation* in changing your lifestyle. We don't just ask, "How can we make your itchy eyes feel better?" We go further and ask, "How can we get rid of whatever is making your eyes itch in the first place?" What you will find in this book is not a one-size-fits-all miracle cure and not a recipe of superficial changes that you can toss away after a week. It is a *total makeover* of yourself and how you approach your allergies, environment, lifestyle, and health.

The good news is that these simple changes will help you for the rest of your life. They will support and strengthen you every day, promoting your physical well-being, eliminating allergy symptoms, and increasing your body's innate healing powers. By following the 7-Day Allergy Makeover, you will get to the root of your allergies so that your body can heal from within, restore its immunity, and eliminate the symptoms once and for all.

> These simple changes will help you for the rest of your life.

Second, we don't treat symptoms with drugs. You will not need any creams, steroids, or shots to feel better. Instead, by naturally eliminating allergens, your body will feel healthy and be better able to deal with life stressors. The book lays out action-oriented, step-by-step instructions on uncovering the root cause of allergies and makes simple but specific changes that can stop the symptoms from recurring. By eliminating the need for drugs, not only do you save money but you avoid potential side effects. In fact, as you will see, sometimes drugs are *part of* the allergy problem, not a solution!

I know firsthand how much pain allergies cause. I know how they get in the way of enjoying life, how they get in the way of work, intimacy, and friendships. Most important, I want you to know that *it doesn't have to be this way.* If you want to support your body's natural healing powers and restore it to its optimal, vibrant state, this book is for you. You can immediately implement the lessons you will learn in this book, and the benefits you feel will last forever.

ALLERGIES DEFINED

Before starting with the strategies for dealing with allergies, we need to take a step back to understand two key concepts. The first is *allergies* and the second is *sympathetic dominance*. Although it may seem self-evident to you what an allergy is (You did buy this book, after all!), a redefinition is in order so that we understand just how deep the problem of allergies runs.

When many of us think of allergies, the first ideas that come to mind are hay fever symptoms such as runny nose and itchy eyes. These allergies often arise from pollen or pet dander. Next, we think of anaphylactic reactions, which can be characterized by a potentially dangerous constriction of the throat and intense swelling. For someone who is severely allergic, this might result from a bee sting or a bite of seafood, egg, or peanuts. Other severe reactions can come from insect bites or a profound allergy to a medication such as penicillin.

This definition of allergies is very helpful. It allows us to identify some of the most severe—and visible—allergic reactions so that we can better treat them. Such reactions are known in the medical community as IgE (for immunoglobulin E) or type I hypersensitivity reactions and are characterized by a noticeable immune response.

How does an allergy manifest? Allergens, or *antigens*, are specific chemical substances (natural or artificial) that are inhaled, contacted, ingested, or injected. Once the immune system detects an allergen, it recognizes it as a foreign substance, and this may trigger a cascade of physiological reactions designed to attack and neutralize that substance. We call the resulting symptoms and processes "allergies" or "sensitivities." Our diet, water, home, and air are filled with countless allergens. They include molds and yeasts, pollens, weeds, grass, chlorine, car exhaust, dust and dust mites, and many types of food.

Yet most allergy tests focus only on such acute—and immediate—allergy responses. If you get immediate inflammation, swelling, and hives, you're probably allergic to the offending agent. But what about a sensitivity reaction to, say, sugar or fluoride? How do we make sense of those? The standard definition of allergies leaves many allergic symptoms—including those that don't produce swelling, constriction, or itchiness—to go undiagnosed.

This book expands the definition of allergies to include a broader range of *sensitivities* or *reactions* to your food, water, chemicals, and environment.

Dr. Susanne's new definition of *allergies/sensitivities*, as used in this book: An allergy or sensitivity is any bodily reaction to nutrients, foods, inhalants, chemicals, or endogenous or foreign substances that produces a cellular dysfunction and disturbs the normal physiology of the cell, gland, organ, or system.

This means it's not just dust mites or peanuts that cause allergies. By this definition, chemicals such as formaldehyde and compounds as common as sugar and plastic also cause dysfunction in your body and, therefore, cause allergies. To me, if eating a certain food causes you to be sluggish and lose concentration, guess what? It's a sensitivity or allergy. I use the two words *sensitivity* and *allergy* interchangeably. These antigens may not give you a typical allergic reaction, such as a rash, or cause your eyes to water, but they prevent your body from thriving at its optimal state, and to me, that's unacceptable. It takes you out of *homeostasis*—the dynamic state of being in balance. Each individual has a unique immune pattern, and how one reacts to allergens/antigens depends on his or her degree of exposure, genetics, overall toxic load, general physical health, and degree and type of stress encountered. Symptoms that the standard definition doesn't account for—constipation, gas, bloating, headache, joint pain, anxiety, insomnia, and fatigue—can cause just as much suffering and frustration in those they afflict. When people come to me to deal with their pollen allergies, they may not even realize that their low energy is caused by eating *wheat bread*. But this is exactly what a more holistic approach to allergies lets us see.

Therefore, according to our new definition, allergy symptoms can be produced by any of the following:

- Fungi (molds and yeasts)
- Pollen, weeds, grass, flowers, trees, resin, natural scents
- Dust, animal dander, dust mites
- Foods (such as proteins found in grains, meat, dairy, eggs, nuts, natural fruit chemicals, red/blue pigments in berries, oils)
- Heavy metals (lead, arsenic, mercury, cadmium)
- Natural nonmetal and metal elements (such as iodine, chlorine, sulfur, aluminum and nickel)
- Chemicals (formaldehyde, toluene and other solvents, polystyrene foam, and plastics)
- Toxins (aflatoxin, dioxin, cyanotoxin)
- Gases (carbon monoxide, propane gas, car exhaust)

SYMPATHETIC DOMINANCE

But there's one other side of allergies that we need to understand: the emotional side. It's very rare to find someone who is emotionally calm who also has allergies. This is not a coincidence. Allergies

> Allergies put us at war with our own bodies.

put us at war with our own bodies. At a primal level, allergens are perceived as "threats" to the body and can create a cascade of fight-or-flight reactions as the body tries to rid itself of these chemicals or toxins. In this situation, your body is not in a naturally relaxed, healthy state because it is struggling for survival! The *sympathetic nervous system* turns on just as it has evolved to do, to deal with emergencies and threats to the body. It fuels itself with stress, and you feel the rush of adrenaline. The more the body fights allergies, the more stress develops. Adrenaline lifts you for a moment, but soon enough, you crash. And this stress creates a vicious circle. The more stressed you are, the more the body wears down from adrenaline rushes, unable to deal with the allergens themselves. In our modern society, mental and emotional issues produced by jobs, obligations, and other external pressures add to this load of stress we carry around. The end result is what we will call *sympathetic dominance*.

Dr. Susanne's definition of *sympathetic dominance*: Sympathetic dominance is a physical state defined by a constant fight, fright, or flight mode, in which the sympathetic nervous system, which is responsible for handling emergencies, begins to control our daily functioning, resulting in emotional wear, adrenal exhaustion, and difficulty in dealing with allergies.

HOW TO USE THIS BOOK

The goal of this book is to help you live an allergy-free life, giving you the opportunity to reach your highest potential—energetically, physically, biochemically, emotionally, mentally, psychologically, and spiritually. You will begin a life transformation in the coming days that will not only help your body but also help you become more generous and free in your life. When you are not struggling with allergies, that time and emotional clarity is yours again. You can then decide how you want to live and what you have to give back to your friends, family, and planet without the weight of your allergies holding you back.

1. Reduce Your Exposure to Allergens

First, I want to teach you how to reduce your exposure to the allergens in your environment. While some allergens may seem quite obvious (for example, car exhaust, mold, and pollen), you are also exposed to numerous *hidden* allergenic substances without even knowing it. Everything from the food you eat to the beauty products you use, to the very air you breathe may carry offending agents. The safest route to living allergy free is to *minimize exposure to all potential allergens*. Reduce the allergen accumulation (toxic overload) within your body, and you'll have fewer symptoms.

The book contains an explanation of many of the most common allergens and the symptoms they can produce. It also gives a complete step-by-step plan for eliminating toxic things from your home and implementing healthy life practices. By following these steps, you will dramatically decrease your overall exposure to allergens, and your body can begin its work of healing.

2. Restore the Body

Second, I want to teach you how to restore and heal your body naturally. Once you begin reducing your exposure to allergens you will replace old life practices with healthful ones, helping your body reach its natural, optimal, vibrant state. Even if you are exposed to as few allergens as possible, you can make changes to your diet, environment, home, and life practices that will strengthen the body's immune powers. A better immune system means a better ability to deal with allergies. And there's a bonus: The more vigorous your body feels, the more happiness you will experience. The benefits of your allergy makeover go far beyond allergies!

The book demands dedication and even what may seem at the time like difficult life changes. I understand that it can be hard to change habits that you have lived with for a long time. It can feel like parting with an old friend. But if you have suffered from allergies and you are *fed up* with them, the changes this book helps you make will be the beginning to a new life. Some of my suggestions will ask you to invest in new kitchenware and equipment that will help purify your tap water and environment. The initial investment may not always be as budget friendly as you might like. You might have to let go of some foods you enjoy. But your health is at stake. What could be more important than that?

Get as much support as you can from your friends, family, and coworkers. This will help you in the coming weeks, months, and years. Perhaps, along the way, you will struggle to make some of these lifestyle changes. Doubts are normal. Partial progress is normal. But KEEP WITH THE PROGRAM! I know that you *will* feel the difference if you follow it through to the end. Even in just seven days your body will have begun doing its healing work. There will always be time to replace your stainless-steel forks with wooden ones, but the time for saying yes to healing is now! You can be back in control of your physical well-being once again. And there is *nothing* more important than that.

STRUCTURE OF THE BOOK

The book is divided into seven days—seven chapters—each focusing on a different aspect of your health and environment while showing you clearly how these contribute to your allergies. I urge you to read each day sequentially. Each day, implement as many of the strategies for allergy health as you can. If Day 3 suggests that you change your air filters, buy an air purifier, dehumidify your closets, and keep the windows shut throughout the day, try to do all these things on Day 3. But if you can't, no worries. Take care of what you can (say, dehumidify the closets and keep the windows shut), and make progress toward your other goals. You might research air purifiers and call someone to change your filters. That's fine! If you can't make *any* progress one day, try to plan out your schedule so that you know *when* you will implement the tools in this book. If you can't buy the air purifier today and just don't have time to look on the Internet, make sure you commit to researching them tomorrow. In the end, this makeover will be as effective as the dedication and energy you put into it. But whether it takes you seven days or seven weeks, follow the guidelines in each chapter. Have patience with yourself, and keep moving forward. I know that if you follow through with everything laid out in this book, you will feel a new life and vigor you haven't felt in ages.

THE SEVEN DAYS: AN OVERVIEW

Day 1: Clean Up Your Nutrition

Your nutrition is a key element in reducing your allergy symptoms, increasing your tolerance, and improving your body's defenses. In this chapter, you will learn about some of the most common (and some surprising) food allergies and the symptoms they produce. You will get tips on what kinds of foods to eat and how they help you with your allergies.

Day 2: Clean Up Your Water

You will learn about the water in your home and how it may be contributing to your body's toxic load. By improving the quality of water in your home, you will reduce your exposure to chemicals and gases that contribute to allergy symptoms.

Day 3: Clean Up Your Air

You will understand how airborne allergens from outside permeate your home, car, and office. The steps outlined in this chapter will help you minimize the staying power of such allergens in the home and help you breathe easier throughout the day.

Day 4: Clean Up Your Living Environment

It is crucial to keep our homes as safe and allergen free as possible. In this chapter, we will discuss dust, mold, and other allergens that originate within our living environments, how they affect your body, and the ways to minimize them in the home. This chapter also has a special section on children's bedrooms and which items can cause the most common pediatric allergies.

Day 5: Clean Up Your Kitchen

The kitchen has more allergens than almost any other room in the house. In this chapter, we'll look at what they are and how to reduce your exposure to them. By properly cleaning and preparing your food as well as eliminating toxic cooking items, you will greatly improve your overall allergy health.

Day 6: Clean Up Your Body

Cleansing practices are an often-overlooked aspect of our overall health. The amount of allergens that collect in our hair and on our body can be astounding. This chapter will detail which cleaning products are safe and healthy, and outline cleansing techniques to eliminate toxins.

Day 7: Clean Up Your Stress

Emotional health is important in reducing your sensitivity not only to events but also to potential allergens. This chapter will explain in more detail the crucial concept of *sympathetic dominance*—the body's reliance on a fight, fright, or flight mode—and how it makes us allergy-prone. You will learn a series of easy-to-practice techniques aimed to calm the body and return our awareness to the present moment.

NOW WE BEGIN

Before we go any further, take a look at the Allergy Symptoms Checklist below. I want you to fill it out so you can clearly identify what problems you are having. Once you have done that, it's time to see how you can benefit from seven days of problem solving that will change your life. I have also added my Body Composition Tracking Sheet, which I use in my office for body measurements and photos to track physical improvements. "Before" and "after" body measurements are helpful if you have abdominal bloating, water retention, fat-loss resistance, or poor muscle development. Before and after *photos* are helpful when you have acne, hives, skin fungal infections, eczema, or any other visible signs of allergies.

So right now, before you read another word, please take a few moments and fill out the Allergy Symptoms Checklist. Simply rate the severity of your allergy symptoms on a scale of 1 to 10 (1 for mildest and 10 for severest) so you can compare them to how you feel after you've completed the program.

Go to the resources section on page 262 to find a link to my website where you will be able to download the Allergy Symptoms Checklist to print. In fact, the resources include a complete list of all charts, checklists, and videos that will be available to you online to support you on your allergy makeover and health journey.

The Allergy Symptoms Checklist

Please fill out this form before and after the 7-Day Allergy Makeover to compare changes in allergy symptoms.

Check any of the following symptoms you may experience and, if applicable, rate them on a scale of 1–10, with 1 = very mild and 10 = very severe. The total refers to the number of symptoms found in each bolded category, not to the severity.

DIGESTIVE TRACT				
❏ Nausea and vomiting		❏ Belching or passing gas	
❏ Loose or pasty stool		❏ Stomach pain or cramps	
❏ Diarrhea		❏ Heartburn or acid reflux	
❏ Constipation		❏ Blood and/or mucus in stools	
❏ Bloated feeling			
			TOTAL	

JOINTS AND MUSCLES

❏	Pains or aches in joints	❏	Swollen, tender joints	
❏	Arthritis	❏	Growing pain in legs	
❏	Stiffness or limitation of movement	❏	Gout	
❏	Pain or aches in muscles	❏	Fibromyalgia	
❏	Feeling of weakness or tiredness			
			TOTAL	

HEAD

❏	Headaches	❏	Facial flushing	
❏	Faintness	❏	Facial numbness	
❏	Dizziness	❏	History of head trauma	
❏	Insomnia, sleep disorder			
			TOTAL	

SKIN

❏	Acne	❏	Hair loss	
❏	Itching	❏	Flushing or hot flashes	
❏	Hives, rash, dry skin			
			TOTAL	

EYES

❏	Watery or itchy eyes	❏	Red, swollen, or sticky eyelids	
❏	Bloodshot eyes	❏	Bags or dark circles under eyes	
			TOTAL	

EARS

❏	Itchy ears	❏	Reddening of ears	
❏	Earaches, ear infections	❏	Excess ear wax	
❏	Ringing in ears	❏	Ear tubes	
❏	Hearing loss	❏	Drainage from ears	
			TOTAL	

NOSE

❑	Stuffy nose		❑	Hay fever	
❑	Postnasal drip		❑	Sneezing	
❑	Chronically red, inflamed nose		❑	Excessive mucus formation	
❑	Sinus problems				
				TOTAL	

MOUTH AND THROAT

❑	Chronic coughing		❑	Swollen or discolored tongue, lips	
❑	Frequent clearing		❑	Canker sores	
❑	Swollen tongue, teeth marks on side of tongue		❑	Itching on roof of mouth	
❑	Sore throat, hoarseness, loss of voice		❑	Gagging	
				TOTAL	

WEIGHT AND APPETITE

❑	Binge eating or drinking		❑	Water retention	
❑	Craving certain foods		❑	Lack of appetite	
❑	Hungry in the middle of the night		❑	Feeling of fullness	
❑	Compulsive eating		❑	Excessive weight	
				TOTAL	

ENERGY AND ACTIVITY

❑	Apathy, lethargy		❑	Restless leg syndrome	
❑	Attention deficit		❑	Poor physical coordination	
❑	Fatigue		❑	Low libido	
❑	Insomnia		❑	Stuttering, stammering	
❑	Hyperactivity, restlessness		❑	Slurred speech	
				TOTAL	

EMOTIONS

❑	Mood swings		❑	Unwarranted fear	
❑	Anger, irritability, aggressiveness		❑	Feelings of overwhelm	
❑	Anxiety, nervousness		❑	Frustrated, cries often	
❑	Argumentative		❑	Depression	
				TOTAL	

MIND

❑	Poor memory		❑	Difficulty completing projects
❑	Confusion		❑	Difficulty with mathematics
❑	Easily distracted		❑	Difficulty making decisions
❑	Learning disabilities		❑	Poor/short attention span
❑	Underachiever in school		❑	History of brain trauma
				TOTAL

LUNGS

❑	Chest congestion		❑	Persistent cough
❑	Asthma bronchitis		❑	Wheezing
❑	Shortness of breath		❑	Air hunger
❑	Difficulty breathing		❑	Sleep apnea
				TOTAL

HEART

❑	Irregular or skipped heartbeat		❑	Heart murmur
❑	Rapid or pounding heartbeat		❑	Valve disease
❑	Chest pain			
				TOTAL

UROLOGICAL/GENITAL

❑	Genital itch or discharge		❑	Enuresis (bedwetting)
❑	Yeast infections		❑	Anal itching
❑	Frequent or urgent urination		❑	Hemorrhoids
❑	Frequent bladder infections			
				TOTAL

OTHER

❑	Frequent illness		❑	Antibiotics as a child
❑	Vaccine reactions		❑	Eat fish/seafood more than twice a week
❑	Mercury fillings			
				TOTAL
				GRAND TOTAL

BODY COMPOSITION TRACKING SHEET

Name:	Weight (lb.):	Height (in.):	BMI: weight ÷ height × 703
Main issue(s):		Pulse rate (bpm):	Blood pressure (mm Hg):

Measurements:			
		Before	After
1. Biceps *(upper forearm)*			
2. Chest *(level with nipple line)*			
3. Waist *(level with belly button)*			
4. Hips *(level with pubic bones)*			
5. Thigh *(3 inches below pubic bones)*			

Photos: include photos of before and after	
Before	Before
After	After

DAY 1

CLEAN UP YOUR
NUTRITION

We start with nutrition for a good reason: Nothing can do as much to reduce the frequency and severity of your allergy symptoms as avoiding the wrong foods. Our immune system is geared toward fighting off toxic things and substances that enter our bodies. So what enters our bodies several times every day? That's right: food. If you think about it, starting here makes a lot of sense.

When patients come into my office, I take a detailed medical and lifestyle history and run appropriate blood, stool, saliva, and urine tests. After I have all of the patient's diagnostic information, I use my medical detective skills to get the holistic big picture of what is happening. That leads me to the root cause of the allergy symptoms. If I see a red flag for peanut intolerance, for example, I go through their entire diet, helping them recognize how they are exposed to peanuts and peanut by-products and start them on a diet that is completely peanut free. Once my patients learn not to eat certain foods, most of them experience fewer allergy symptoms, and increased energy and vibrancy, by the end of the very first week! Typically, after a month, the allergy symptoms have disappeared altogether. My patients come back and tell me they are delighted and feel so much better, and usually they are amazed at what was causing the problem in the first place.

Most people do not realize the crucial role the digestive system plays in fighting off allergies. Your immune system is not contained in an organ located in some mysterious place inside your rib cage. Rather, it's made up of special cells, proteins, and tissues spread throughout the body, which defend it against invasions of disease-causing agents such as microbes, heavy metals, and toxic chemicals. More than half the immune system lies in your digestive tract, because we eat most of the "foreign" agents that enter the body every day.

One of the immune system's primary defenses is the nearly five pounds of bioflora in your intestines. These bacterial "good guys" not only fight harmful bacteria, fungi, and parasites but also form a barrier on the intestinal wall so that harmful germs cannot enter the blood and lymph systems. If spread out, this intestinal lining, or wall, would cover an entire basketball court! The healthy bacteria aid in the digestion process of food and fiber and optimize the assimilation of the vitamins and minerals into your bloodstream to nourish your body. But when you eat too much of the wrong foods, take too many antibiotics, or are exposed to heavy metals and toxins, you can develop what is known as leaky gut syndrome. The unhealthy gut barrier causes intestinal permeability (in other words, it "gets leaky"), causing undigested larger molecules of food and proteins to enter the bloodstream, which in turn triggers immune system agents to recognize the allergens and attack those molecules. That, in a nutshell, is why you need to avoid food that will provoke these attacks.

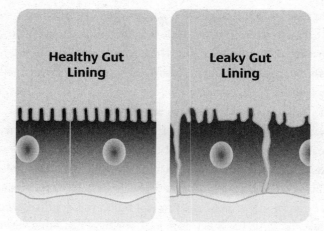

For anyone reading this book, I recommend that you have some diagnostic tests done.

Genova Diagnostics has a valuable Intestinal Permeability Assessment to check for leaky gut. Basically, the test involves you to swallow two substances: lactulose and mannitol. Before and after urine tests will indicate whether you have a leaky gut. If you have a healthy digestive mucosal barrier, these two substances will stay in the gut and pass out with your bowel movements. But if you have a positive intestinal permeability, or leaky gut, then these two substances will pass through the leaky gut lining, get filtered out through the kidneys, and show up in the urine. The reason for the two types of substances is to help indicate what size particles are able to pass through the gut mucosa. The more lactulose found in the urine, the larger the pore size in the gut lining. The more mannitol and less lactulose found in the urine, the smaller the pore size. This will help your doctor determine the course of the gut restore program, or which nutritional supplements will heal your leaky gut. Not all doctors are familiar with this test, so you may need to give the information to your physician so he or she can order it for you. For more information on the intestinal permeability test, check the resources section of this book. And if you want to learn more about leaky gut syndrome—and how it might be compromising your digestive health—there is an article available on my website.

Food allergy testing methods are also readily available, though somewhat limited in their reliability and accuracy. Trained medical doctors commonly perform two types of food sensitivity tests. The skin prick test is conducted by placing a drop of prepared solution containing the food allergen, usually on your back or forearm. The second commonly performed test is a blood test (radioallergosorbent test, or RAST). Both tests look for hyperimmune reactions to foods by measuring the IgE levels. These tests can be useful, but 50 to 60 percent of the results give false positives, so they are far from definitive.

Some food allergies are hidden and are difficult to detect because the reactions are more latent—it takes more time for the symptoms to appear, and they often are ambiguous and easily mistaken for some other health concern such as headache, insomnia, foggy brain, or fatigue.

IgE-mediated allergic responses are immediate and are easily detected with overt symptoms such as hives, runny nose, or itchy eyes, whereas in latent allergy reactions measured by IgG level (immunoglobulin G differs from IgE), symptoms may not occur for hours, and may take 24 or even 72 hours to appear.

A number of clinical laboratories are now conducting these latent food allergy tests, which measure IgG-mediated allergenic responses. These tests use ELISA (enzyme-linked immunosorbent assay) methodology.

Some doctors and other health practitioners are strong proponents for these tests, but I find they can be costly, may not be covered by insurance, and are prone to producing false positives. False positive results are usually due to a cross-reactivity phenomenon. This happens because some food families have very similar protein strands, which can mimic another type of allergenic food. The person being tested may not truly be allergic to the food that indicated a positive result; instead the test triggered a similar reaction due to the similar protein strand.

Stool tests are also available to test for gluten sensitivities by Genova Diagnostics and EnteroLab.

The gold standard of food allergy testing is the food elimination methodology.

Here is how I approach each allergy patient: Identify all allergy symptoms; pinpoint allergenic triggers through history and testing; prescribe my allergy-free dietary protocol by eliminating specific allergenic foods; implement my allergy makeover program; and after a few weeks, reevaluate the symptoms list and see the difference. The drawback here, of course, is that it does take time and patience.

You may find, though, as many of my patients have, that your doctor just wants to write a prescription. If you do not feel any better after taking the medication, this is the perfect time to try my allergy elimination diet and finally get to the *root causes* of your symptoms.

I should point out that many of my patients become wary when they hear the words *elimination diet*. Yet the process of restricting what you eat does not mean you have to eat green beans every night for the rest of your life. I advise people to eat a balanced amount of protein, vegetables, oils, and the right types of carbohydrates. You are not going to starve from trying to cure your allergy. You will simply learn how to choose foods that make your body healthy and less reactive. Having fewer sensitivities means you are promoting a healthier immune system.

In the appendices, you will find a shopping list full of healthful allergy-reducing foods. The list includes suggested vegetables, grains, fruits, legumes (beans and peas), and meats that you can buy to fill up your refrigerator and pantry. The food list provides plenty of delicious alternatives to the foods you are consuming right now that are making you sick.

I will add one extra point that covers all the food allergies: You do need to be honest with yourself. This is not the same as being on a diet. In that case, if you sneak a handful of chocolate-covered peanuts, you may not be able to reach your target weight goal as quickly. You tell yourself, *I'll be good tomorrow*. But food sensitivities/allergies are different. Your body needs four days to neutralize and detoxify allergens and antigens. Even if you eat the food that causes an allergic reaction as little as once every four days, you will *still* experience symptoms constantly, without any break at all.

By following the simple steps in this chapter, you'll start to feel better right away. You can help yourself the most by *controlling what you put into your body*. Let's find out what different types of foods might be contributing to your overall symptoms right now. That's the first step in starting to feel a whole lot better.

> Your body needs four days to neutralize and detoxify allergens and antigens.

CLEAN UP YOUR NUTRITION IN 6 STEPS

Step 1: Eliminate Allergenic Foods/Beverages from Your Diet

You eat food primarily to nourish and maintain a healthy body, but sometimes your body may not agree with *what* you are ingesting.

Many of these foods can cause a true allergic reaction, but I have also found in my practice that eating certain types of foods can cause reactions that merely produce discomfort. For example, someone may not have a true wheat allergy, but eating cereal products gives her headaches. Many people are lactose intolerant, but that doesn't mean, in strict medical terms, that they are allergic to milk. With food, the primary issue is, how are you feeling after eating your favorite meal? Do you feel energized, or tired? Are you able to focus on a project, or do you have difficulty concentrating? Can you help yourself feel better?

Here is a list of seven foods and beverages that many people are sensitive to, even without knowing it:

- Dairy products
- Gluten grains
- Sugars
- Fungi (molds and yeasts)
- Alcohol
- Eggs
- Peanuts

Remember, not all these will trigger IgE (or acute) allergic symptoms. But over time, they can wear down your immune system. Let's look at each food category to better understand how they may be contributing to your illnesses.

Dairy Products

The first food type may come as a surprise. For years, we have watched advertisements that promote how healthy milk is for you. It has calcium that helps you build strong bones, not to mention being a good source of protein. So we should drink three glasses of milk a day, right?

An entire food industry has been built around dairy products. These include milk and milk derivatives such as cheese, yogurt, frozen yogurt, and ice cream. Yet milk can also be found in many other products that you might not suspect. Certain salad dressings, pasta sauces, and even chips and other baked goods may contain dairy products. Although butter comes from milk, it mainly contains fats, so it doesn't create as many allergy problems. That's because butter usually doesn't contain the three main culprits that produce adverse reactions: *lactose, casein,* and *whey.*

I should point out that eggs are often mistaken as a dairy product, but that isn't correct. They may come from the same farm the milk comes from, but there the similarity ends. Eggs come from chickens, ducks, and other animals that lay eggs, and none of these is a dairy-producing animal. Eggs are a different form of food allergen that we'll talk about later on in this chapter.

So why do dairy products produce bad reactions? It's because, after you are five years old, your digestive organs stop producing the enzymes that break down what are called *macromolecules* in milk, such as lactose and milk proteins. Undigested milk then enters the intestinal tract, where your gut's immunity and bacteria start reacting to it, causing discomfort and symptoms. Why does our body stop making those enzymes? The fact is, the human digestive system has not evolved to process cow's milk. Mind you, this is the *perfect* drink—for baby cows. Not only are we drinking the milk of another species, but we are the only mammals that drink milk as adults, which leads to a variety of health problems. A major reason for these problems is that cow's milk is designed to help

> The human digestive system has not evolved to process cow's milk.

calves develop to maturity, when they will weigh roughly thirteen hundred pounds. We don't grow to anywhere near that size.

The tremendous amounts of bovine growth factors added to cow's milk are another huge issue. Unless the carton says organic, the dairy industry relies heavily on growth hormone additives that keep the milk flowing in cows. Antibiotics are freely used to prevent infections. Pesticides are sprayed on the feed. You may be sensitive to more than just the natural ingredients in milk. You may also be reacting to the hormones and chemicals injected or fed to the cows. Remember, our immune system fights off what it deems to be foreign substances in our body, and that immune reaction is what produces most of your allergy symptoms.

People have a right to be confused. We're told that dairy products are good for us, but it turns out they can contribute to our illnesses. Luckily, information is power. So let's take a look at the symptoms and see if any of them fit how you feel.

SYMPTOMS. There are two basic health issues associated with dairy products. The first is known as *lactose intolerance*. Many people know or know of someone with this condition. So what does it mean? Lactose is a milk sugar made up of two simple sugars that are bonded together: glucose and galactose. The enzyme lactase, which is found in the small intestine, is required to break lactose down into the two simple sugars for proper absorption. After infancy, most of us stop producing the lactase enzyme. The lack of that enzyme makes us sensitive, to varying degrees, to dairy products. The most common symptoms of lactose intolerance are diarrhea, nausea, abdominal cramps, bloating, and gas. People of African, Asian, and Latin American descent have a higher likelihood of lactose/dairy sensitivities due to their genetic heritage.

The second problem is directly related to allergies. Cow's milk contains two proteins that can cause an allergic reaction. Casein, which is found in the solid part (curd—the part of milk that curdles), is considered an excitotoxin, which is known to overstimulate the nervous system. Casein can produce anxiety and insomnia in some people. With children, overconsumption of casein may lead to hyperactivity associated with attention deficit disorder. When you are looking at an ingredient list on a food package, look out for other names of casein. These include ammonium caseinate, calcium caseinate, magnesium caseinate, sodium caseinate, and rennet casein.

Whey, which is in the liquid part that remains after milk curdles, is found in many popular protein shakes. It does provide benefits. It can help build muscle, help immune system functioning, and increase the production of a very important antioxidant called glutathione. But it can also cause many allergy symptoms due mainly to two types of dairy proteins, called α-lactalbumin and β-lactoglobulin. In addition, whey also has lactose as an ingredient. Many people who have dairy allergies experience gas, belching, constipation, weight gain and difficulty losing weight, skin rashes, eczema, acid reflux, diarrhea, acne, abdominal cramps, yeast infections, excess nasal secretions, and more. By the long list of reactions to dairy products, you can see why I have put it at the top of my food allergy list. It is *the* leading cause of the problems I see in my patients.

Action item. Eliminate all dairy products from your diet containing lactose, casein, and whey. The list includes all milk products made from cows, goats, sheep, buffalo, and yak (yes, yak!). These animal milk products are found in milk, cheese, ice cream, and yogurt as well as salad dressings, sauces, packaged foods, beverages, protein shakes, milk chocolate, cheese-flavored tortilla chips, and pastries made with dairy ingredients. Read the ingredient list on the package thoroughly. Beware of these substances: *sodium*

Not Ready for the Beach

Eczema is a skin condition in which the sufferer has patches of rash that are itchy and very dry. These patches are red and can ooze fluid when scratched. A fourteen-year-old girl named Emily came into my office. Her mother said she had suffered from eczema since soon after birth. Her case was severe, meaning that many areas of her skin were affected. She had huge patches inside her elbow, on the back of her elbow, in the crease behind her knees, and on her breasts. Half her scalp was thickened and scaly, causing a constant rain of dandruff. She had gone to numerous doctors, who prescribed topical drugs for her skin. At this age, when children are so self-conscious, she had to wear long-sleeved shirts and long pants throughout the Southern California summer. Emily would not wear a bathing suit because she was so embarrassed by her rashes.

When I inquired about her diet, I found that she had some form of dairy food at every meal. She would have milk with her cereal, cheese on her omelets. She said she absolutely loved cheese. After conducting tests, I told Emily she had to give up all forms of dairy, which was very difficult for her. I asked her to replace the dairy products with almond milk, along with dairy-free, casein-free cheese. Sure enough, after a few days, she began to notice that her eczema patches were not as itchy. After two weeks, she could see a clear difference, and after a month, she found that she didn't need the topical drugs anymore. She really started coming out of her shell because she no longer had any reason to be ashamed of her skin. She was so happy with her body, she started wearing shorts, short dresses, tank tops—and bathing suits.

caseinate and *calcium caseinate*—they are commonly found in popular alternative cheese products, but they're dairy by-products. If you decide to use butter, ghee (clarified butter) is the best choice. Avoid these dairy foods, and see if your condition starts to improve.

Before you start to worry about how you can possibly do without a glass of milk, you should know that a whole host of nutritious and tasty alternatives can substitute for dairy products. Milk alternatives are now made of rice, almond, hemp, and coconut. Many supermarkets now carry soy milk, but be sure to buy organic, non-GMO (genetically modified organisms) soy milk. Soy, rice, and coconut nondairy yogurt, ice cream, and casein-free cheese are sold at all health food stores and even by some supermarket chains. These products also substitute well in cooking recipes and are included in the shopping list in the appendix. As with all the foods in this chapter, you can make yourself feel worlds better merely by being a smart shopper.

RESTAURANT TIPS. How can you protect yourself when eating out? Most restaurants are very accommodating if you tell your waiter or manager that you are allergic or sensitive to dairy products. Here are some simple steps you can take:

- Ask for rice milk, almond milk, or soy milk instead of half-and-half or milk for your tea or coffee. (I carry a small carton of my own organic almond milk to restaurants.)
- Ask for oil-and-vinegar dressing instead of ranch dressing. (Balsamic vinegar and olive oil is a popular choice.)
- Hold the cheese on your omelets, tacos, burritos, burgers (served without the bun), beans, soups, salads, appetizers, and so on.
- Ask for a dairy-free soup of the day.
- Have fruit or sorbet instead of ice cream.

Gluten Grains

Many people around the world rely on wheat as a staple. Foods such as white bread, pasta, whole-wheat bread, pizza, hamburger buns, sandwiches, pastries, cookies, cakes, pancakes, and even soy sauce are made with wheat. Wheat flour is even used in candy snacks such as red licorice sticks commonly sold in movie theaters. It can seem to be in every meal you eat!

Yet we as a species have not always eaten wheat. Before the first agricultural revolution (roughly ten thousand years ago), humans were hunter-gatherers. Cereal grains were not part of the Paleolithic diet, because they are produced mostly by farming. Our ancient forebears' food sources consisted of wild meats, fruits, seeds, nuts, and vegetables. So in terms of our genetic heritage, wheat is a recent addition to our diet. More important, our immune system doesn't always accept it—and that can mean allergies.

Gluten is a naturally occurring protein in wheat that makes the dough elastic and sticky. But gluten is also found in many other cereal grains, including rye, barley, triticale (a cross between wheat and rye), and other varieties of wheat, including spelt, kamut, bulgur, semolina, farro, and durum. Oats are naturally gluten free but are frequently contaminated with wheat during farming and processing. But gluten's seeming omnipresence doesn't end there. It is used as a binding agent and can be found in a diverse array of products, including certain medicines, vitamins, lipsticks, and even stamps.

You may have noticed all the "gluten-free" cookbooks that have been popping up lately. What is gluten-free, and who needs to avoid gluten? Nearly three million Americans have celiac disease, a serious autoimmune condition caused by severe gluten intolerance. These individuals must keep to a purely gluten-free diet for life. Special blood tests and biopsies can provide a definite diagnosis of celiac disease.

There are three IgA (immunoglobulin A) blood tests for celiac disease that detect the levels of gluten autoantibodies. These are EMA (anti-endomysial), TTG (anti-tissue transglutaminase), and DGP (deamidated gliadin peptide). For these tests to be accurate, the patient needs to be on a gluten-containing diet. A more aggressive evaluation of the gut lining involves a surgical procedure in which a small bowel biopsy is made to assess damage to the gut.

There Are Three Types of Gluten Sensitivities

- **Gluten intolerance** occurs when your small intestines lack the enzymes to digest the gluten proteins. It can cause functional digestive symptoms such as gas, bloating, constipation, and other irritating symptoms such as headaches, joint pain, and anxiety. Physiological reactions are temporary, and symptoms will go away if you eliminate the offending agent (that is, gluten).

- **Gluten allergy** occurs when your immune system has an overreaction to the specific gluten protein. It can trigger IgE-mediated allergic reactions, such as rashes, hives, and itching, as well as even more serious reactions, such as wheezing and difficulty breathing. This type of reaction can be fatal, so the allergic person may need to carry an EpiPen for emergency response to anaphylactic reactions.

- **Celiac disease** is an autoimmune condition caused by permanent gluten intolerance. The immune system generates an abnormal response to ingested gluten foods and attacks the small intestine's lining, causing cellular damage, malabsorption of nutrients, and other serious complications.

Even though we may not have severe celiac symptoms, many of us are sensitive to gluten in some way. Even if you test negative on all three gluten autoantibody blood tests (EMA, TTG, and DGP) for celiac disease, you could have a condition known simply as *gluten intolerance* or *sensitivity*. Whereas only 1 percent of the population has celiac disease, a study has found that gluten-reactive patients may make up as much as one-tenth of the population. If

Missing in Action

Laura, a thirty-five-year-old woman who looked anorexic when she first came to see me, had symptoms that baffled medical science. She had seen five different doctors, who had prescribed two MRIs, a colonoscopy, an endoscopy, and barium x-rays, among other tests. What were they looking for? She had severe pains and cramps in her stomach. She also had acid reflux, bloat, constant fatigue, and severe constipation, meaning she went as long as a week at a time without having a bowel movement. Sadly, she had three young children but was in such pain that she could not handle the duties of being a mother.

Although she did not suffer from celiac disease, a gluten-sensitivity stool test indicated that Laura was extremely reactive to gluten grains. I advised her to stop eating all products containing gluten. Within a few days, the first sign of her recovery was to have a bowel movement without needing laxatives. She started gaining weight because she was feeling less and less pain in her stomach. Her acid reflux went away. Within four weeks, *all* her symptoms, including the fatigue, had disappeared. She started to exercise regularly and now she is very active with her children.

you have any of the symptoms listed in the following section, you should try to go wheat or gluten free. You may find that you feel a real difference!

SYMPTOMS. Gluten allergy symptoms range from mild (such as itching, hives, runny nose) to severe (such as difficulty breathing and anaphylactic reactions). If you are gluten intolerant and have difficulty *digesting* foods containing gluten, this causes a negative reaction and a host of other symptoms. The most common include cramping or pain in the stomach or abdomen, acid reflux, constipation, diarrhea, inflammation or joint pain, fatigue, cold hands and feet, headaches, foggy brain, and even anxiety and insomnia. If you experience any of these symptoms, I highly recommend reducing or, preferably, eliminating your intake of wheat and other gluten grains.

Action item. Foods containing gluten include bread, crackers, pasta, bagels, soy sauce (tamari is okay), white and whole wheat flour, oats (unless specified as gluten-free), barley, rye, spelt, farro, and triticale. If you are experiencing allergy symptoms, start clearing these items out of your kitchen cabinets. Consider donating them to a local food bank or homeless shelter.

I am well aware that this step can seem like a real sacrifice, because gluten grains make up a huge part of the American diet. The good news is that they can be replaced with a whole array of other grains. Some are available at any supermarket, and you can find others at a health food or ethnic food store.

Recommended replacements for gluten grains are brown rice, wild rice, corn (non-GMO, if you please), gluten-free oats, quinoa (pronounced *KEEN-wah* and eaten as a grain though it's actually an herb seed), and amaranth. Although white rice *is* gluten-free, I don't recommend it, due to its high sugar content and low nutritive value. White potatoes fit basically into the same category as white rice; a starch that spikes your sugar level. Alternatives to gluten grains are included in the shopping list in the appendix. Many health food stores carry gluten-free breads, pastas, and pastries, which are often made from rice flour, nuts, and other ingredients. Read all labels, even packages from health food stores, and be mindful of the number of grams of sugar per serving. Coconut, almond, sweet potato, chickpea, and brown rice flour can be substituted in many baking recipes.

Although beans and sweet potatoes are not in the grain family, both can be a great substitute as a healthy carbohydrate alternative to gluten grains. As with dairy products, at first the task seems daunting. Yet, as all those people buying gluten-free cookbooks have found out, once you start thinking about the wide variety of foods that taste just as good and can fill you up the same way, you simply move your hand one foot farther down the supermarket shelf and put different items in your shopping cart!

RESTAURANT TIPS

- Ask the waiter *not* to bring the basket of bread.
- Tell the waiter you are gluten and wheat sensitive, and ask about hidden gluten, often used in gravies, sauces, and soups.
- Look for gluten-free carbohydrates such as sweet potato, brown rice, beans, corn tortillas (non-GMO), brown rice noodles, polenta, roasted potato, quinoa, amaranth, hummus, butternut squash, organic tofu, and gluten-free oats.

Sugar

Everyone loves sugar. Some of my patients confess that they are addicted to it. Others say they cannot live without a bite of chocolate every day. Sugary foods and beverages such as sodas, cookies, candy, and sweetened coffee are often the first choice when we need a quick jolt of energy. Delicious treats such as cake, ice cream, and sweetened pastries tempt us at every turn. And yet we all know what we're getting when we consume too much sugar: loads of calories but absolutely no nutrients.

Sugar also produces a yo-yo cycle of highs followed by lows that makes us feel tired and irritable. Sugar from outside the body raises the blood sugar inside the body. A surge of glucose sugar gets dumped in your bloodstream, triggering the pancreas to release a rapid surge of insulin. Insulin is a hormone that helps even out your high blood sugar level and helps deliver blood glucose to your various tissues and organs—muscles, liver, brain, and so on. These rapid surges can be dangerous to your health. As time passes and your body keeps experiencing constant high and low swings of your blood glucose levels, you increase your risk of diabetes. In 2011, an estimated 25.8 million children and adults in the United States—8.3 percent of the population—had diabetes, and that number is climbing!

So when I speak of sensitivity or an allergy to sugar, I do not mean that you are actually experiencing an immune reaction. I am addressing the dangers of our body's reaction to constant jolts of sugar, which can lead to lower energy levels, brain fog, anxiety, and lethargy.

Many of my patients are confused about the different types of sugar. Is sugar produced by the sugarcane or sugar beet plant the same as the sugar in fruit? Fruit contains sugar, and we all know that fruit, up to a point, is good for you—full of vitamins, antioxidants, minerals, and fiber. (I say "up to a point" because too much fruit can cause fatty liver and increase allergy symptoms.) The best way to explain why all sugars are not created equal is to sum the difference up in one word: *fiber*. Fiber in food is vitally important because it slows down carbohydrate digestion in the gut and helps regulate how fast your blood sugar levels rise.

Most sugary foods or drinks that we consume, however, are

lacking fiber. Those are made with refined sugar. That means they are not natural. The fiber has been refined out of the food. Most of the sugar we consume consists of either table (cane or beet) sugar or high-fructose corn syrup, which the food industry uses in a wide variety of products. Candy and most sodas are extremely high in refined sugar. Most breakfast cereals also contain a lot of refined sugar; in fact, in some, refined sugar is the *main* ingredient! Most cookies, cakes, pies, and ice cream also fall in the high-sugar category. This list can't be all that surprising to you. They aren't called "sweet temptations" for nothing.

Finally, artificial sweeteners can also be considered sugars. Studies have found that people who use artificial sweeteners actually *gain* weight instead of losing it. Moreover, artificial sweeteners are synthetic chemicals and have been shown to cause allergic reactions and various physical ailments.

As long as we are discussing spikes in your blood sugar levels, you should be aware that they can also be caused by foods that don't contain refined sugar. Your blood sugar can be sent sky-high by foods containing starches, particularly simple carbohydrates such as most white grains and flours (white wheat flour, white pasta, white rice), which have had their fibrous elements removed, and starchy vegetables such as white potatoes.

There is some confusion about carbohydrates, so I'll give a simple explanation. Carbohydrates ("carbs," for short) fall into two basic groups: simple and complex. The difference between the two is based on their chemical structure and how quickly we digest and absorb them. Simple carbohydrates are either a single sugar molecule (monosaccharides) or a slightly larger molecule made up of a short chain of two monosaccharides (disaccharides).

Complex carbohydrates are made of three or more sugars linked together, forming a chain of sugars. The longer molecules are digested more slowly because the body has more links to break.

That slower process of digestion can keep the blood sugar from rising rapidly. Complex carbs include vegetables such as pumpkin, sweet potato, and eggplant; grains such as quinoa and brown rice; legumes such as lentils and black beans; and nuts such as walnuts and almonds. These foods also have plenty of fiber. Again, notice that fiber can be a great help in keeping our body on an even keel. Not only are these foods digested slowly but they are also packed with vitamins and minerals. So the type of carbs you want to avoid are the simple carbohydrates. All the cookies, pies, cakes, and pastries I mentioned before are also simple carbohydrates.

A useful guide for judging how fast a food raises your blood sugar after eating is the glycemic index (GI). GI is a ranking of carbohydrates on a scale from 0 to 100. Foods with a high GI (over 55), such as white sugar, white rice, white flour, and white potato, are digested and absorbed quickly. They raise the blood sugar rapidly, followed by a quick rise in insulin from the pancreas. On the other hand, low GI (below 55) foods are digested slowly, producing a gradual rise in blood sugar and insulin levels. To find the glycemic index ranking of foods, either search "glycemic index" online or go to the University of Sydney's GI page (glycemicindex .com) to find a complete list. All of the recommend foods in the Allergy-Free Food Shopping List on page 247 are considered low glycemic index.

There's one more important part of the sugar equation: What if you have trouble digesting sugars?

Many people are intolerant of foods replete with what are known as "fermentable carbs." These include fructose, lactose, galactose, xylitol, and sorbitol. Foods that are high in such fermentable carbs are called "FODMAP" foods, which stands for fermentable oligo-di-monosaccharides and polyols. Gluten grains, dairy products, and alcohol are all high-FODMAP foods, which is yet another reason to avoid them. But so are beans, lentils, and peanuts; many healthful vegetables, such as cabbage, cauliflower, and broccoli; and fruits such as apples, pears, peaches, and nectarines. These foods can create digestive issues such as bloating, gas, diarrhea, constipation, and abdominal pain. Some 20 percent of Americans have the same symptoms that go with a diagnosis of irritable bowel syndrome (IBS). IBS can be debilitating, painful, and unpredictable. Although the root cause of IBS is still a mystery to the medical profession, I have found that 75 to 80 percent of my IBS patients find relief by avoiding these special sugars and by reestablishing a healthy gut flora.

The reason the body has a difficult time processing such fermentable carbohydrates is that we do not produce the right kind of digestive enzymes to break special sugars down. Instead, these are largely dealt with in the gut by bacterial fermentation, a natural process that extracts the maximum amount of energy from them. The end result of the fermentation process is gas, which usually stays within levels the body can tolerate.

But when your gut bioflora is thrown off—by stress; the ingestion of antibiotics, heavy metals, and toxins; or an overgrowth of unfriendly bacteria—these sugars can feed the bacteria, producing an excess of gas buildup. This can result in bloating, abdominal pain, and constipation, or it can have an osmotic effect, rapidly drawing water into the gut, causing diarrhea. It's horribly uncomfortable and unpredictable and can be a real drain on your energy.

By avoiding high-FODMAP foods, IBS symptoms will subside, and you will also help reduce the excess bacteria just by starving them. If you want to heal your gut allergy symptoms, you will have to avoid these foods as well—temporarily. For a comprehensive list of high-FODMAP foods to avoid and low-FODMAP foods to eat, please refer to my Gut Restore Food Checklist on page 252.

If you believe you have an irritable bowel, here's what you can do to start helping your gut heal. Begin simply by following my allergy makeover protocol as outlined in this book, particularly eliminating gluten, dairy, alcohol, and refined and artificial sugar from your diet. If, after two or three weeks, you notice some change but not a considerable difference in your IBS symptoms, begin the low-FODMAP Gut Restore plan for four to six weeks.

This will require you to pay a little more attention when you shop. An easy way to do this is just to look over the beneficial low-FODMAP Gut Restore food list on page 252 and stick to those items. You can also go to the resources section for the URL to print out the entire FODMAP Gut Restore chart for easy consultation. There are many delicious low-FODMAP foods, such as quinoa, brown rice, meats, blueberries, raspberries, grapes, carrots, arugula, eggplant, red bell peppers, and chard.

After four to six weeks, if you start feeling better, begin introducing probiotic foods, such as miso soup, kimchi, sauerkraut, and nondairy yogurt to your diet (about twice a week), to build up good gut bacteria. At that time, you still may wish to continue to limit your exposure to high-FODMAP foods such as beans, broccoli, apples, and cabbage, if you find you have a particular sensitivity to them.

SYMPTOMS. Sugar sensitivities are extremely common and often contribute to feelings of brain fog, lethargy, irritability, dizziness, anger, muscle cramps, fatigue, anxiety, restlessness, and insomnia. Sugar intolerance symptoms include abdominal bloating and cramping, flatulence (gas), belching, feeling of fullness, acid reflux, and constipation or diarrhea.

Excess sugar intake also reduces the concentration of potassium inside the cells (which is vital for the cells to function properly). And it causes water to move out of the cell, into the extracellular tissues, leaving the body dehydrated at the cellular level and making you feel terribly thirsty. People who eat a lot of sugar and sim-

All Without Ritalin

I had a patient named Alex, a kindergartener who was terribly hyperactive. He whined all the time, and his mother said he had difficulty concentrating at school. Alex couldn't follow instructions from his parents or his teacher. He couldn't even dress by himself. When I examined and evaluated his diet, I quickly realized that his daily food intake was just *filled* with sugar. Adding to the problem, he loved any food that was white: white bread, snacks made of white flour, pasta, rice, and potatoes. So I prescribed an allergy elimination diet: no sugar or starches for him.

Because Alex's parents ate the same way their son did, I had a hard time changing his diet at first. It took three months of urging them before they finally took my advice. Slowly but surely, rather than eating take-out meals, the family started to cook more at home and added more lean protein and vegetables to their diet. They followed my directions to change his school lunch menu as well. Instead of a peanut butter and jelly sandwich with orange juice for lunch, he got turkey meatloaf with carrots and celery sticks and a bottle of purified water. The more Alex's parents kept up with the sugar-free diet, the more his cravings for sweets shifted and decreased. With a more stable blood sugar level throughout the day, Alex became more attentive in class. He stopped throwing temper tantrums. Rather than venting his frustration in physical displays, he became more verbal, telling his parents how he was feeling. At school, he stopped disrupting the class. Ultimately, his parents realized that it wasn't fair to sit down to dinner with him and eat the foods he used to love but could no longer have. They had to change their diet, too. As a result, the entire family ended up improving their health.

ple carbohydrates usually look swollen and bloated from the water retention in their tissues. I always ask my patients to show me their tongue so that I can look for the telltale sign of an excessively sugary carbohydrate diet: a swollen, fat tongue that has indentations from the teeth along the sides.

Action item. If you really check out the ingredients, you'll find that many processed foods, especially soda, candy, and cereals, contain refined sugar, such as table sugar, honey, molasses, agave, corn syrup, maple syrup, and synthetic sugar substitutes. The most common food items containing starches are white bread, white flour, white pasta, white rice, white potatoes, jams and jellies, cookies, pastries, dried fruits, and juice. Try to reduce your consumption of sugar at the same time you clear out your pantry—if sugary foods aren't right there on hand, you won't be so easily tempted.

The three natural substitutes for sugar are stevia, made from the sweetleaf plant; xylitol, a naturally occurring sugar alcohol found in fibers of fruits and vegetables; and erythritol, a sugar alcohol found in fruits and fermented foods. These taste a bit different from refined sugar, but they will give your organic tea or baked items a sweet taste without raising your blood sugar level. If you have irritable bowel issues, it's best to use stevia and erythritol only; xylitol can cause gas, bloating, and loose stool.

Many people who crave sweets may actually need to add more protein to their diet. Check to see if your current diet contains enough meat, fish, legumes, seeds, nuts, high-protein grains, and vegetables. A typical serving of meat is about the size of a deck of cards. For most meals, your plate should contain about one-fourth protein (four to six ounces), one-fourth complex carbohydrates, and one-half vegetables. Integrating more beans, lentils, wild-caught fish, grass-fed beef, chicken, or eggs (if you don't have sensitivities or irritable bowel symptoms) can be a great way to cut the sugar cravings and balance out your blood sugar.

You will find a complete list of proteins in the shopping list on page 247. Meal portion sizes are discussed in step 5, later in this chapter.

RESTAURANT TIPS

- Choose foods with a low (below 55) glycemic index (foods that don't make the blood sugar level fluctuate rapidly).
- Instead of a full glass of freshly squeezed orange juice, ask for a quarter glass of juice mixed with carbonated water.
- Drink herbal tea instead of a vanilla-flavored latte.
- Carry stevia, xylitol, or erythritol packets with you for your organic tea or coffee.
- Order fresh fruit instead of your favorite pie à la mode.

Fungi (Molds and Yeasts)

If you have respiratory allergy symptoms that do not abate even when hayfever season is over, you may be allergic to the mold and mold spores in the environment. Mold spores are prevalent everywhere in nature, including on your foods. (We'll talk about how to minimize mold buildup on your food in step 2, later in this chapter.) But let's not forget that many of the foods you eat *are* fungi or have mold in them. This class of allergens includes all mushrooms as well as food products made with yeast, particularly bread products. Also included are foods that contain mold, such as some cheeses. The blue-green veins in blue cheese (including Roquefort, Gorgonzola, and Stilton) are actually live *Penicillium* mold (the source of the drug penicillin!). Wine and beer, in addition to containing yeasts, are also contaminated with molds. In scientific terms, ethyl alcohol, or ethanol (the alcohol in wine, beer, and liquor), is considered a mycotoxin—a by-product of fungal fermentation, the process whereby yeast converts sugar into alcohol.

Because so many forms of mold are airborne, occur naturally in soil, and grow on the surfaces of living organisms, you also need to watch out for foods that harbor molds and their spores. Molds and slime molds readily accumulate on many vegetables, fruits, and salad greens and must be washed properly before eating. The same precautions need to be made to avoid the mold, slime mold, and spores that accumulate on cheese, dried fruits, nuts (peanuts, cashews, pistachios), and, often, packaged snack food items, including fruit and nut bars.

Choked Up on the Podium

One day, James, a forty-two-year-old with a stressful job as one of the top leaders in the tech industry, came in to see me. He had a chronic cough, along with a postnasal drip that made his voice sound nasal. This condition was a real problem because he was in the media a great deal, giving interviews and lectures, and he constantly had to clear his throat during his speeches. He had had the condition for more than a year and had seen the best doctors and clinics in the country.

After I conducted a detailed history and evaluation we discovered that he was eating foods that were contaminated with molds, especially the blue cheese on his salads. He also ate loads of greens in restaurants, and he didn't know that most restaurants don't wash their greens, but buy it in big bags from farmers.

We eliminated these foods from his diet, and within two weeks, his cough and his postnasal drip disappeared. He is loving his new, clear voice much better than the old nasal one!

Finally, molds can grow excessively in any nonfrozen packaged food such as crackers, potato and corn chips, grains (both bulk and packaged), and especially rice. To learn how to wash rice, fruits, and vegetables properly, ridding them of molds, bacteria, and debris, see page 162. Ideally, you should reduce your use of packaged food products.

SYMPTOMS. Many people who are sensitive to fungi may experience the following symptoms: a tickle in the throat, sore throat, headache, itchy skin, bloating, immediate hives, a swollen tongue or cold sores, abdominal pain and cramping, fatigue/ lethargy, red eyes, nasal congestion and runny nose, joint pain, frequent urination, irritability, anxiety, and insomnia. In my practice, I find that many of my patients have an underlying fungal infection that contributes to their chronic illnesses. By eliminating fungi from your diet, you may be pleasantly surprised at how many troublesome issues clear up in a short time.

Action item. If you think you may be allergic to mold, you need to consider all products containing yeast. These include bread, bagels, doughnuts, crackers, brewer's yeast, and any soup base made with autolyzed yeast extract. You should also examine the following products that likely contain mold: mushrooms, wine, beer, dried fruits, peanuts, peanut butter, cashews, pistachios, cheeses, fresh berries (it's difficult to find a box of berries without mold contamination unless they're frozen), and nonfrozen packaged food products (anything in boxes, plastic bags, or wrappers).

RESTAURANT TIPS

- Ask the waiter to omit all mushrooms, peanuts, cashews, and cheese from your meal.
- Avoid dried fruits in salads and other dishes.
- Order fresh fruit without the berries and grapes. Pass on the bread basket.

- Instead of a green salad, order steamed, sautéed, roasted, or grilled vegetables.

Alcohol

Many of us love to have an after-hours drink or a glass of champagne on special occasions. Some people have a glass of wine or beer with dinner. But if you are suffering from allergies, even an ounce of alcohol can contribute to your long-term issues by wearing down the body's defenses.

A host of health problems are associated with alcohol consumption, including impaired judgment and decision making, blood sugar spikes, insulin insensitivity, and increased anxiety, lethargy, and brain fog. But let's not forget about alcohol's role in allergies.

The oxidation of alcohol (ethanol) inside the body produces acetaldehyde, thought to be one of the contributing factors of a morning hangover.

People have allergic reactions to drinking because alcohol triggers a release of histamines, which are natural substances produced by the immune system. Histamines play a major role in many allergic reactions in the body. They stimulate blood vessels to dilate, decreasing blood pressure, they cause gastric juices to flow, and they also cause constriction of lung tissues. High concentrations of histamines are also found naturally in plants as well as in by-products of bacteria and of yeast fermentation in beer, wine, and liquor.

In addition to histamines, beer and wine also contain sulfites. These are used as a preservative but can also provoke respiratory distress, headaches, nasal congestion, and other irritating allergy symptoms.

I should also point out that eating too much fruit can create what I call "autointoxication," or "autobrewery." Fruit, combined with yeasts and molds in your intestines, can cause alcohol fermentation in the gut, which increases allergy symptoms and may even make you feel as though you had a hangover. So be mindful, and limit your intake to one or two pieces of fruit per day.

Party Girl

Jessica was a twenty-eight-year-old single lawyer working in a very stressful law-firm environment. She told me she went out three or four nights a week with friends and for work functions and had one or two glasses of wine. The next day, she always woke up with fatigue, brain fog, headaches, and pain in the lower-right ribs. A physical evaluation revealed that the tenderness was located right over the liver area. Blood tests showed high levels of liver enzymes, and her sugar was in the higher range of normal. I investigated further, and she confessed that she also took Tylenol daily for her headaches. She also drank more than she first told me: more like three or four glasses of wine and often an after-dinner drink as well.

I strongly recommended that she cut out her drinking and taking painkillers. Both were contributing to her liver disease. In this case, I also asked her to take some time off work so she could deal with the detox symptoms. I supported her with supplements to ease her detoxification and to heal and rejuvenate her liver. After three weeks of cleansing, the headaches and the pain in her liver subsided. Her brain fog cleared up, and she had enough energy to exercise, which helped keep her work stress in check. After four weeks, we retested her liver enzymes, and the levels were completely normal. She also slept better, had more energy, and was more productive at work. She had quit drinking altogether and didn't miss it.

SYMPTOMS. Alcohol-sensitive individuals may have symptoms such as acid reflux, indigestion, nausea, itchy red skin, nasal congestion, joint pain, headaches, anxiety, brain fog, migraines (especially after drinking red wine), insomnia, and difficulty losing weight.

Although alcohol poisoning is rare, if you have a severe allergy to alcohol it can be fatal. That's because the liver has a difficult time processing alcohol. Thus alcohol consumption contributes to your overall toxic burden, making it difficult for the body to properly process the chemicals. If you have allergies to vinegar, you can have severe reactions after ingesting alcohol.

East Asian people are also known to have a genetic predisposition to an enzyme deficiency that causes difficulty in breaking down alcohol and its derivatives. This intolerance can cause red flushing of the face and chest, rapid heart rate, nausea, and even alcohol poisoning.

Action item. Because alcohol, like sugar, is so tempting, it's best to clear the house of all products containing alcohol if you have an alcohol sensitivity. This will help you eliminate or at least limit alcohol intake. If you do decide to drink, nongrain vodka, tequila, and sake should be considered the better choices, because they are free of extra allergens such as sulfites and mold.

For more information on ways to feel better naturally—such as taking more time for yourself and being in the present moment—see "Day 7: Clean Up Your Stress," on page 210.

RESTAURANT TIPS

- Order sparkling water and add lime, mint, cucumber, or watermelon for a refreshing taste and go alcohol-free.
- Instead of wine or beer, add one ounce of gluten-free vodka, tequila, or sake in a tall glass of ice with sparkling water. You can add lemon, lime, mint, cucumber, or watermelon.

Peanuts

We have all heard of someone who has experienced potentially life-threatening reactions from eating peanuts. You don't even have to eat them to have a reaction. Some people are so sensitive to peanuts that even a tiny dab of peanut oil or the smell of a friend's peanut butter sandwich can cause problems.

Most peanut allergies are a hypersensitivity to a specific strand of proteins in peanuts. People with this allergy have to take extra precautions. While avoiding peanuts seems easy to do, many factories make other products on equipment that also processes peanuts. So if you are sensitive, please, *always* check the back of the box for allergy warnings.

I should point out that peanuts and peanut butter can easily be contaminated with molds and mycotoxins (toxic substances produced by a fungus) because of the way the peanuts are processed. Peanuts are not true nuts at all, but part of the legume (beans and peas) family. And like beans, peanuts come from a pod. When they are being dried, moisture from the pod can promote mold growth that ultimately becomes toxic. I am pointing this out is because some people believe they are reacting to peanuts when, in fact, they are sensitive to the mold.

SYMPTOMS. Peanut allergy symptoms can include hives, rashes and swelling, itching, tingling or swelling around the mouth and throat, abdominal pain, diarrhea, vomiting, shortness of breath, and wheezing. If you have any symptoms that are possibly life threatening, such as swelling of the throat and tongue, this can lead to anaphylactic reactions. These are severe reactions that can result in hospitalization and even death. In this case, you must carry an EpiPen (an injectable medicine that will open up your airways in seconds) at all times. After using the EpiPen, get medical attention immediately.

Action item. Acute peanut allergies are serious business. You

No More PB and J

Amanda complained that she had a hard time waking up in the morning. She needed an alarm clock to get up by nine, and she had to start her workday after noon because she couldn't clear her head and body until then. I took a full history of her diet and found out that she ate peanut butter—lots of it—twice a day. When I say "lots of it," I mean she went through a jar of it every four or five days. I told her she needed to stop eating peanut butter because of the allergenic effect as well as the possible exposure to a mycotoxin called *aflatoxin*, which is common in peanuts and peanut butter. Upon hearing my advice, she started to cry. She said she was addicted to peanut butter. I suggested several alternatives, including almond butter, hazelnut butter, and sesame tahini, and although she wasn't happy about it, she was willing to try.

Sure enough, after two weeks of going peanut free, she came into my office—for a 10:00 a.m. appointment, no less—full of energy and raring to go. She said she was waking up at 7:00 even without an alarm clock. She had energy to burn, enough that she could see more clients and expand her business.

must clear your house of *all* peanuts, peanut butter, peanut oil, and foods that may contain peanuts. Check the labels of all foods, including cereal, crackers, and ethnic dishes. If you have severe reactions to peanuts, you're better off not eating *any* types of nuts and seeds, due to the potential for cross-contamination at the manufacturing plant. Read all labels!

But even for those without a severe allergy, it's wise to avoid peanuts—not because they are bad in themselves but because of the increased risk of mold contamination.

Luckily, you can find many nut and seed butters at any health food store. These include almond, macadamia, hazelnut, hempseed, and sesame seed butters. Like peanuts, cashews also can have excess mold growth, so if you find you have allergic symptoms after eating peanuts, it's best to steer clear of cashews, too.

RESTAURANT TIPS

- Ask if any of the dishes include peanuts, and if the chef can't leave them out, order something else.
- If you have severe reactions to peanuts, call the restaurant in advance and ask if they use peanuts, peanut oils, or peanut butter in any of their dishes. If so, find another restaurant.

Eggs

Most people eat eggs in some form every day: two- or three-egg omelets, pancakes made with eggs, French toast, egg bread, egg-battered chicken, real mayonnaise, Caesar dressing. Eggs are not usually thought of as provoking allergies, but they are actually one of the most common allergies for children. These reactions can be quite severe, as was the case with my son. Anytime he had so much as a bite of food containing eggs he would immediately have swelling in his throat, difficulty breathing, and hives all over his body. If you are breastfeeding, you should be aware that if you consume eggs, your infant may have an allergic reaction to egg proteins in your breast milk. Once a child reaches the age of six these reactions usually subside, but even with adults, eggs can be a hidden allergy and difficult to diagnose.

> Eggs can be a hidden allergy and difficult to diagnose.

Children with egg allergies have to be very careful when receiving childhood vaccines. Two common childhood immunizations—the MMR and flu vaccines—may contain egg or egg-related proteins that can cause mild to severe allergic reactions. In addition, vaccines for travelers, such as those for yellow fever and typhoid fever, also contain egg-related proteins.

SYMPTOMS. Egg allergies can produce eczema and red, itchy rashes, stomach troubles such as cramps and nausea, or even symptoms similar to those of hay fever: itchy eyes, runny nose, and asthmatic reactions. Severe egg allergies may cause anaphylactic reactions, in which the inflammatory reaction can be aggressive and block the airways.

Arthritis Begone

Symptoms of egg allergies can be insidious. Robert, a forty-two-year-old patient complained of joint pain in his fingers. They were slightly swollen but not red or painful to the touch. The pain and stiffness occurred when he moved the fingers, stretched out his hand, or clenched his fist. Because his father had arthritis, he thought it was just part of getting older, and routine testing didn't provide any conclusive results.

He decided to try the 7-Day Allergy Makeover. He wasn't all that eager to give up so many of his favorite foods, so we began slowly removing the allergens. Every third day, we removed another, starting with dairy, then gluten grains, sugar, and so on. Within two weeks, he reported a 30 to 40 percent improvement. Then we found the biggest culprit: he was eating three to four omelets a week and usually an egg salad sandwich for lunch. Once we eliminated eggs, his joint pain and stiffness completely disappeared within four days.

Action item. People with this allergy need to be careful about eating any fresh eggs, Caesar and ranch dressings that contain eggs or mayonnaise, pastries made with eggs, any frozen items breaded with an egg batter, egg bread, pancakes and waffles, and any other foods containing egg yolks or egg whites.

As for alternatives, as long as you aren't sensitive to soy products, organic tofu is a great replacement for scrambled eggs in the morning, especially if you add turmeric and other spices. Depending on the recipe, you can use tofu with ground flaxseed or other all-natural egg substitutes found in the health food store. For sweet recipes, bananas, sweet potato, or pumpkins will often do the trick.

RESTAURANT TIPS

- Ask if any eggs or egg products are used in your favorite meals.
- Instead of eggs and bacon for breakfast, ask for turkey bacon and roasted tomatoes, or gluten-free oats if available.
- Use balsamic or lemon vinaigrette dressing instead of Caesar dressing.
- Use vegan mayo instead of real mayonnaise.

Step 2: Add Plenty of Fiber to Your Diet

Fiber (cellulose) is a crucial part of the 7-Day Allergy Makeover diet, even though it's a type of carbohydrate that the body can't digest. As fiber passes through the gut it helps remove waste from the body. It binds up toxins and other chemicals in your system so they can be eliminated. It also promotes the growth of beneficial bacteria in your intestinal tract and promotes optimal bowel move-

> When food is processed, its natural fiber is broken apart.

ment frequency (at least one or two per day). You can think of it as a scrubber that works inside your tubes.

The recommended daily intake of fiber is 35 grams. The problem is, most Americans consume only about 5 grams, leaving them sorely deficient in fiber. That's because we eat so much processed food. When food is processed, its natural fiber is broken apart. For instance, in the manufacture of white flour, the sifting breaks apart the protective outer layer of the bran, which holds fiber. White rice is processed as well because the outer husk is removed. That's why eating more unprocessed foods, such as vegetables, beans, nuts, seeds, and whole grains will help you get a healthful amount of fiber every day.

TWO KINDS OF FIBER. Fiber comes in two kinds: soluble and insoluble, and both have beneficial effects on your digestion.

Soluble fibers dissolve in water, forming a gel-like substance that makes you feel full, slows down digestion, and can help control weight. Here are some common sources of soluble fiber:

- Oatmeal and oat bran
- Lentils
- Apples
- Pears
- Nuts
- Flaxseed, chia seeds
- Beans and dried peas
- Cucumbers, celery, and carrots (carrots have both soluble and insoluble fiber)
- Glucomannan and psyllium (natural fibers in foods and supplements)

Insoluble fibers add bulk to the diet, helping prevent constipation by stimulating bowel regularity. These fibers are not water soluble, so they pass through the digestive system relatively intact. Their bulk speeds up the peristaltic action (smooth muscle contractions) of the bowels. Insoluble fibers are found mainly in whole grains and vegetables. Here are some common sources of insoluble fiber:

- Whole grains (brown rice, corn bran)
- Seeds (sesame, pumpkin, sunflower)
- Nuts (almonds, hazelnuts)
- Zucchini, celery, green beans
- Broccoli, cabbage
- Onions, tomatoes
- Carrots, cucumbers
- Dark leafy vegetables, such as collard, kale, and chard
- Fruit

You will also find all these high-fiber foods in my Allergy-Free Food Shopping List on page 247.

I should note that as you increase the amount of fiber in your diet you may experience more intestinal gas. Remember the discussion of FODMAPs in the sugar section? High-fiber foods can also be high-FODMAP foods. If you have irritable bowel symptoms, be sure to avoid high-FODMAP foods (check the appendices). You should add fiber gradually and drink plenty of purified water to help the soluble fibers do their job.

Action item. Shop for foods containing both soluble and insoluble fiber. If you read the labels, most of them specify the amount of fiber, in milligrams, in each serving. You can also find online many charts that list the amount of fiber for each food.

Wound Up Too Tight

Willa, a high school senior, reported that she had been constipated for five years. She attended a very competitive all-girls school and was feeling a great deal of stress over college applications. She had only one bowel movement a week unless she used laxatives. The teenager was thin but had a swollen abdomen, along with abdominal pain and flatulence (gas). She exercised every day and had a low-calorie, very low-fat diet consisting mainly of protein (chicken, egg whites, fish) and some vegetables (green beans, spinach, broccoli).

I immediately asked her to add more insoluble fiber to her diet—brown rice, zucchini, onions, tomatoes, carrots, cucumbers, kale, and fruit—because insoluble fiber acts as a natural laxative and adds bulk. I also recommended soluble-fiber foods such as beans and gluten-free oats to increase the water content in her stool. Her flatulence resulted from excess undigested protein, so I advised her to eat her meals slowly and chew each bite at least twenty times. I reduced the excess protein in her diet by a quarter and added more healthy fats: nuts and seeds, avocado, and olive oil.

I recommended that she reduce her exercising to three times a week. She was already stressed enough with her schoolwork, and by exercising daily she was constantly in a "sympathetic overloaded state," which prevented her body from relaxing enough to initiate a bowel movement. I also gave her relaxation techniques to practice.

She followed my advice (albeit reluctantly), and within a month, she started to have normal bowel movements four or five times per week, without the use of laxatives. Moreover, she loved her flattened stomach and how her energy level shot up. She also noticed that her feelings of stress had reduced dramatically. Toxins, microbes, and waste that used to sit in the gut were now being eliminated regularly, and that restored her energy. Needless to say, she is enjoying her transformation!

RESTAURANT TIPS

- Order a variety of vegetables, beans, and gluten-free grains with your protein meal.
- Add chia seed and flaxseed or almonds to your favorite dishes.

Step 3: Cook and Clean Foods Properly

Despite recent trends toward raw-food diets, cooked foods provide many advantages for allergy control. Cooking foods eliminates bacteria and fungi as well as viruses and parasites. You should, however, use proper cooking equipment (glass, iron, or enamel pots and pans) to avoid ingesting chemicals and metals found in plastics, nonstick aluminum, and stainless-steel pots and pans. Recently, there has been some excitement about "green" ceramic cookware, but some studies are showing that specific brands of noncoated ceramics can be contaminated by heavy metals.

A detailed explanation of proper food-handling techniques and kitchen organization is provided in "Day 5: Clean Up Your Kitchen."

When eating raw foods, it is vital to clean them properly, as they may harbor mycotoxins, bacteria, fungi, and parasites. You should wash and peel all appropriate fruits because peels often collect mold. For fruits that aren't peeled, such as organic grapes, strawberries, raspberries, and blueberries, you should buy vitamin C crystals or powder from a health food store and wash the fruits as outlined on page 162.

Action item. Soak and wash all fruits and vegetables with vitamin C powder. Peel all fruits and vegetables, when appropriate, and cut off all areas of bruising (fungal fermentation).

Step 4: Eat Whole, Organic, Locally Grown Foods in Season

These days, we buy strawberries grown in Spain, avocados from Mexico, and rice from Japan. While globalization has produced many benefits for consumers, the growing and shipping of food have caused a number of problems. The first concerns agribusiness's common methods of growing food. Many people are now aware of the importance of eating organic foods to reduce the intake of pesticides, fungicides, hormones, antibiotics, heavy metals, and chemicals that are sprayed, injected, or fed to what we eat. The toxins and additives are believed to irritate and weaken the gut mucosal lining, contributing to a leaky gut. Undigested larger molecules of food seep through the leaky intestines into the bloodstream, causing aggressive immune reactions and allergy symptoms.

A second concern is the mold that collects on transported food. Even when shipped in from a nearby state, the food may sit in trucks for a long time, encouraging the growth of fungi. Packaged foods can also collect mold in them over time.

Third, foods that have been shipped from distant locations have been scientifically proven to have lower nutritional content than local and seasonal foods. Local foods can be found at farmers' markets, which provide the added benefit of allowing you meet the people who grow your food. Some local farmers let you cut and harvest your own vegetables and fruits. Make a fun outing of it with your family or friends!

You can also sign up for a community-supported agriculture (CSA) program, whereby you buy a weekly share of a local farm's harvest. The growers prepare a box of fruits and vegetables for you each week for pickup (or sometimes even delivery). By buying organic foods, you are also encouraging farmers to grow foods in a sustainable way, while promoting the well-being of their workers. Even if you can't shop at a farmers' market, many stores now indicate where foods are grown, so you can see whether they are local or imported.

How about growing your own organic herbs? It's easy to find potted basil, rosemary, cilantro, parsley, and more at farmers' markets, nurseries, and grocery stores. Grow them indoors in front of a window with good light, and clip off sprigs to add flavor to your meals.

Not only is going organic good for minimizing allergies but eating local foods will also lower your carbon footprint. Transporting food to your local grocery store consumes oil. Spraying crops from planes consumes oil. Making fertilizer for industrial crop production consumes oil and degrades the soil. The less we demand items from beyond a hundred miles from home, the less often supermarkets will order those foods.

And let's not forget organic meats and eggs. At my local farmers' market, there is a farmer who comes down from northern California every Sunday to sell grass-fed, antibiotic-free, hormone-free frozen beef and pork. By meeting the owner personally and talking to him about his farming techniques, I know that I am providing clean and healthful meats for my family. I actually have to preorder my favorite—oxtail, for my Korean oxtail soup—because it is always the first thing to sell out!

Action item. Buy organic foods whenever possible. Look online for the locations and times of your local farmers' market as well as community-supported agriculture programs. Find local farms you can visit and where you can harvest your own fruits and vegetables. Create your own organic herb garden. Look for meat vendors at your farmers' market, and ask how they raise their cattle, hogs, and chickens and whether they are grass fed and drug free.

RESTAURANT TIPS

- Frequent restaurants where chefs buy sustainable and organic produce and meats from local farmers. Many are proud to advertise where they get their food.
- Order meals made with seasonal vegetables and fruits.

Step 5: Eat the Right Proportions

Now it's time to chow down! Pick up your fork out and let's begin.

Each meal should contain a balance of protein, vegetables, healthful carbohydrates, and fats. While the ideal amount will vary by person, the following works well for most individuals:

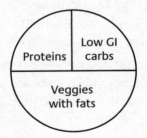

- Vegetables fill half your plate.
- Protein fills only a quarter of your plate (4–6 ounces, the size of a deck of cards).
- Low-GI carbohydrates (gluten free) fill the last quarter (½ to ¾ cup).

- Add small amounts of healthy fats: one to two teaspoons of oils, nuts, or seeds.

Emphasizing that vegetables should fill half the plate may come as a shock for many people, but considering the amounts of vitamins and nutrients they contain, it's astounding that we don't eat more. No single step will do more to help your cells remove toxins and eliminate allergens.

In determining the amount of protein per serving, unless you are a competitive athlete or bodybuilder, a typical portion of meat should be about the size of a deck of cards (four to six ounces). Oils and fats from meat are sufficient for your fat needs, but we all need variety, so add small amounts of healthful oil to your meals (olive, sesame, or coconut oil) or other whole food fat sources (seeds, nuts, avocados).

Finally, remember that vegetables add to your quota of complex carbohydrates, so if you eat a lot of veggies, don't eat an overabundance of grain carbohydrates, which can lead to a host of problems including blood sugar imbalances, weight gain, and fatigue. Keep gluten-free grains under three-quarters cup per meal, but don't eliminate them altogether. Complex carbohydrates are essential for maintaining healthy adrenal gland function, balancing your energy level, calming your nervous system, and optimizing deep sleep.

Step 6: Chew Each Bite of Food Twenty Times

Want to know a very easy way to reduce your allergies? *Chew your food.* Most of us live in or near a fast-paced urban environment, where everyone is in a rush to eat their meal and get back to work, study, or play. Many people inhale their meals within ten minutes. "Eating" in this case is less about chewing than about swallowing

The Parts of Your Plate

Zack, thirty-five years old and overweight, was six feet tall and weighed 230 pounds. Even though he exercised four times a week, he wanted to lose 30 pounds of fat, not muscle. He was a muscular man with an apple body shape and substantial belly fat. Looking over his daily food journal, I learned that he ate three times a day plus a snack, but he ate way too much at each meal. His breakfast consisted of four eggs, pork sausage or bacon, and toast. His portion of a steak was twelve to sixteen ounces—that's three or four servings for an average person. He ate four or five rolls at dinner and drank at least two beers every night. For lunch, he had either a turkey-and-cheese sandwich or a cheeseburger—no veggies.

The answer to his problem was simple: He needed to learn portion control. I told him one serving of meat should be the size of a deck of cards, or four to six ounces of protein. He then had to fill half of his plate with veggies—steamed, grilled, or baked. I told him to ditch the bread and add a half cup of beans, sweet potato, or brown rice. We used two eggs and two egg whites instead of four whole eggs for his omelets, served along with spinach, avocado, green onions, and cilantro. He switched to chicken sausage or turkey bacon instead of greasy pork products. Tomato slices replaced toast. I also added one extra meal to stop the cravings that made him eat too much at dinner.

The first week was brutal for him, but he came back to the office 7 pounds lighter—1 pound lost every day. After four weeks, he had lost 15 pounds. After two and a half months, he had achieved his goal of 200 pounds—his weight in college. He needed to buy new, slim-fitting clothes because everything was too loose on him. He also mentioned that his intimate life with his wife had gotten more fun, and that was a big plus!

mouthfuls of food. How can we digest our food for proper nourishment if we wolf it down so fast?

If you don't chew your food, you don't digest it properly, and that alone can contribute to food allergies. Improper digestion taxes the system and reduces the amount of nutrients you derive from your food. Undigested food also feeds the harmful bacteria and fungi in the intestines, causing bloating, gas, constipation, and diarrhea. Indigestion is often a symptom of not chewing properly.

Chewing twenty times each time you take a bite facilitates the digestive process by releasing enzymes in the mouth and saliva. Breaking larger molecules down into easier-to-process ones helps you properly absorb the nutrients you are taking in. Also, by taking more time to eat your meal, you let your body catch up, and it will feel full before you've ingested the entire plate of food.

To start, count the number of times you chew each bite. Slow down and enjoy your food—really experience how good it smells and tastes. Conscious eating is better for your overall health, and your meals will be more delicious. It's also a great time to practice mindfulness—simply being in the present moment while you eat—which can help reduce your stress level (discussed in detail later in the book). After a while, chewing more thoroughly will become second nature.

Action item. This week, count the number of times you chew each bite. Keep counting as you work your way up to twenty times.

Day 1 addresses an extremely important cause for many allergies. Your body simply may not be able to tolerate what you are putting on your plate. As with any new diet, doubts and concerns may arise. There are a couple of articles on my website that may help you address two of the most common issues with special diets—feeling like you don't know what to eat and how to get your family on board with your new eating plan. Once you have rearranged your diet, though, you need to consider how you can prevent other sources of allergies from making you miserable. At this point, let's move on to another part of your life that is closely related to food: water. Once you understand the problems related to Earth's most precious resource, your health will take another crucial step forward.

DAY 2

CLEAN UP YOUR
WATER

In this chapter we focus on cleaning up the water in your home because it is one of the largest contributors to inflammation and allergy symptoms that I have seen in my twenty-four years of clinical experience.

I was born in Seoul, South Korea, in 1962, the Year of the Water Tiger, and I lived there until I was twelve years old. I have vivid memories of my early childhood, and to this day I am struck by just how different my life was back in Korea—especially in how I think about water.

Some of my favorite memories were the weekend visits I took to my *halmoni*'s (grandmother's) home. When I was two years old, as soon as I could take simple directions, she taught me how important bathing was to my health and made it a part of my daily ritual. Every weekend, we would walk with our toiletries in a bucket to a local bathhouse and spend at least two hours chatting with the neighborhood ladies and cleaning our bodies.

Remember, this was Korea in the 1960s, so water was a very precious resource.

Halmoni's bathroom was basically a porcelain hole in the floor. That's it—no plumbing, no flushing, no sinks or showers. My aunt spent hours each week flushing the waste away with countless buckets of water, and I grew up realizing just how precious running water is.

We were lucky, however, because Halmoni's apartment did have two sources of running water: one outside in the courtyard and one in the detached kitchen just near her living space. But running water didn't mean *clean* water.

All day long, the stoves were loaded with pots of water, the air thick with steam, just as in my *uhmuhni's* (mother's) kitchen. Pots of boiling water were carefully taken off the stove and their contents left to cool. It was the daily ritual of boiling water to make it safe to drink.

Back then, I think just about every household in Korea boiled water because it was filled with bacteria, viruses, and parasites. During my whole time in Korea, I don't remember a single instance when I drank water directly from a faucet. Running water simply meant water for washing our clothes and dishes, taking showers, and watering the garden.

Quite simply, there was no such thing as clean, fresh, pure water.

Unfortunately, this is still true for billions of people around the world. The World Health Organization reports that about 2.6 billion people—half the developing world—lack even a simple latrine with plumbing and 1.1 billion people have no access to *any* source of clean drinking water.

In my birth country of South Korea, things have improved. Forty years later, I can say that three-quarters of South Korea's households use a home water purification unit or drink bottled water. But in poor and rural areas of Korea, the people still boil their drinking water to eliminate microorganisms. The daily clang of pots on the stove and air heavy with steam are the norm. While those numbers are encouraging, my country is one of the lucky ones compared to many places in Latin America, Africa, Asia, and the Middle East.

When I emigrated to the United States in 1975, I was amazed that we didn't have to go through the same ritual of boiling our water but could drink it straight out of the faucet. I could never imagine a place where we could make our tea with the same water that we used for cleaning dishes and taking showers.

Here in the United States, we think that, although it may have some traces contaminants, our water is generally safe to drink. We think that most dangerous forms of water contamination have largely been taken care of by concerted enforcement of environmental regulations.

Unfortunately, study after study shows that this is simply not the case. My professional work as an allergy specialist has given me countless examples of patients whose allergies have disappeared within weeks or even days, *simply because they stopped ingesting tap water and started drinking the proper kind of filtered water.* These case studies, which I share with you later in the chapter, along with scientific evidence, have convinced me that along with the food you eat, the water you drink does more than anything else to encourage the cycle of allergy symptoms.

After conducting this research and witnessing firsthand that poor-quality water is a major contributor to the suffering of my patients, I was

> Along with the food you eat, the water you drink does more than anything else to encourage the cycle of allergy symptoms.

forced to ask myself a startling question: When it comes to water, have we really come so far from my childhood days in Korea?

THE TRUTH ABOUT OUR TAP WATER

The sad fact is that the tap water in our country, as in so much of the world, is simply not safe to drink. While no one doubts that developing countries often have the worst cases of water contamination, the water in the United States is filled with microbes, chemicals, and other harmful substances to a shocking degree.

I live in a suburb of Los Angeles, and we get our water from the Los Angeles Department of Water and Power (LADWP). The LADWP puts out an annual report about the quality of our drinking water; I study it carefully.

From the report, I learned that my tap water contains arsenic, uranium, lead, barium, and other toxic chemicals such as trihalomethanes, nitrates, and haloacetic acids. The water even contains fecal coliform bacteria, including *E. coli.*

The first time I read this report, I was shocked. Arsenic? Uranium? Do these really belong in our water? With so many studies examining the effects of acute exposure, it made me wonder why more studies didn't focus on the long-term health and allergy problems created by a lifetime of ingestion of these chemicals in our tap water. Are even *trace* amounts acceptable?

How were all these toxins affecting my health, including my allergies?

Some of these chemicals cause allergic symptoms directly, whereas others are more indirect. It may be surprising to learn that chlorine is one of the worst offenders when it comes to having a direct impact on your allergies. Chlorine is added to tap water to eliminate microbes such as bacteria and viruses. Because of this caustic chemical nature, it can also cause skin allergies. People with chlorine sensitivities usually complain of itchy skin, rashes, and hives. It can also lead to respiratory allergies including coughing, wheezing, and trouble breathing. What's more, chlorine is known to react with other chemicals in the water and produce bromoform in the body (which can lead to sluggishness and brain fog) as well as dibromochloromethane, which has been linked to a variety of cancers. Fluoride, which is discussed in more depth later, can also contribute to skin rashes as well as asthma and other respiratory allergies.

According to a 2012 study, chlorine also has an indirect effect on allergies. Dichlorophenols (often found in herbicides but used for chlorination) are believed to kill beneficial bacteria in the gut. This makes it harder for the digestive system to process many foods and can contribute to food allergies, possibly even anaphylactic reactions. This reduction in gut bioflora via the work of dichlorophenols may be responsible for the rise in food allergies in Western societies.[1] Remember, chlorine is used specifically for its power to kill harmful waterborne diseases, such as cholera, typhoid, and hepatitis A. But that means it can also kill good gut bacteria too.

Should we really be drinking chlorine and fluoride day in and day out if we want to reduce our allergic symptoms?

It is vital for those suffering from allergies to reduce their exposure to gases and chemicals that can have a *direct* or *indirect* impact on allergies.

While most cities meet government regulations for these chemicals—regulations that may not be strict enough when considering the potential long-term health effects—other cities have failed to keep their tap water safe. It's not just people in rural areas or those who pull water from wells who are prone to an acute overexposure to such chemicals but also people in cities such as San Diego, Las Vegas, Houston, and Jacksonville. These cities, considered some of the nation's worst for drinking water quality, have been found to have an excess of trihalomethanes (such as chloroform), arsenic, uranium, and manganese.[2] Even if you don't live in one of these cities, knowledge is power.

I urge you to go online and look at your city's water quality report for yourself. No matter what's in your water, I've found some practical and inexpensive ways to protect yourself and your family from waterborne toxins and allergens.

Clean Water?

There was a time when water pollution in America was almost entirely unregulated. Factories could dump whatever they wanted, whenever they wanted, and extensive lab testing of our water supply was not the norm.

Over time, regulations came about, in large part because of the nascent environmental movement to produce the two most important federal laws in place today: the Clean Water Act and the Safe Drinking Water Act. Although both have done a lot of good to make our tap water generally safer than it was, have they made our water truly allergen free?

The Clean Water Act, passed in 1972, established regulations for dumping pollutants into water sources and tried to prohibit unregulated discharges into our waterways. However, these regulations have not been able to prevent abuses by major polluters. The Environmental Working Group's report "Dishonorable Discharge: Toxic Pollution of America's Waters" claims that from 1990 to 1994, manufacturing and extraction industries "dumped more than a billion pounds of toxic chemicals into America's rivers, lakes, streams, bays and coastal waters," including "30 million pounds of carcinogens."[3] While permitted dumping accounts for part of the story, much of the pollution is illegal. According to the report, illegal dumping poses serious health risks since "most pollution of America's waters is unregulated and unmonitored."[4] The report states that the three most polluted water sources are the Mississippi River, the Ohio River, and the Pacific Ocean, all of which lie within "dumping distance" of many major metropolitan areas.[5] This means that many potential allergens make it into the water without the knowledge of the city or other federal agencies.

And yet not much has changed since 1994. A 2009 *New York Times* article reports that Lisa P. Jackson, then the administrator of the Environmental Protection Agency (EPA), believes that "despite many successes since the Clean Water Act was passed in 1972, today the nation's water does not meet public health goals, and enforcement of water pollution laws is unacceptably low."[6]

These reports really woke me up. Dumping was not something I wanted to be part of. Not only was it bad for the environment but it was contaminating our waterways and, ultimately, finding its way into our tap water and into our bodies, contributing to people's allergy symptoms.

But there's even more to the story. Such direct dumping accounts for only a portion of the overall pollution of our water. Let's not forget about more indirect sources of water contamination, what is known as *nonpoint source pollution*. Nonpoint source pollution means that the contaminants do not come from a specific source, such as a municipal government, factory, or farm, but are left behind on the streets and open lands, usually as industrial byproducts. Motor oil on the road, fertilizers in lawns, chemicals used to wash and wax our cars, bacteria and feces from animals— all this and more is considered nonpoint source pollution.

A wide range of allergens can travel in such runoff: acids, heavy metals that injure gut integrity, pesticides that can deplete gut bioflora and increase food sensitivities, and bacteria that enter the water from farmlands.

The Clean Water Act does not regulate nonpoint source pollution. That means there is no oversight for how much of this ambient pollution is allowed to make its way into our water.

And what happens to the water that doesn't immediately go back into a river, lake, or stream? In urban environments, rain enters the sewers, where it mixes with human waste products. Normally this doesn't pose a problem. But when the sewage system gets backed up, that water overflows and comes rushing forth onto the streets, eventually finding its way into lakes, rivers, or the ocean. And yes, that's nonpoint source pollution.

The microbes from human waste are far from harmless and many can find their way into our tap water. The organization American Rivers reports that the microbes carried in sewage have been responsible for numerous cases of "diarrhea, vomiting, respiratory, and other infections, hepatitis, dysentery, and other diseases," as well as playing a role in long-term diseases such as "cancer, heart disease, and arthritis."[7] And don't forget, consuming bad bacteria can also increase your sensitivity to foods, creating excess gas, constipation, or abdominal pain after eating. Bad bacteria also compete with the friendly bioflora that help ferment food and break it down for maximum absorption. This means that gas buildup and increased sensitivity to many foods—including healthful but hard-to-digest fermentable carbohydrate foods (discussed on pages 46–47) such as broccoli, cabbage, and beans—may be the result of bad bacteria in your drinking water.

In 2012, the destruction caused by Hurricane Sandy moved us as a nation. Thousands of people from around the country contributed financially or directly in the rebuilding process. But unfortunately, the flooding also produced the kind of problems with sewage contamination we have just talked about. If you are in one of the affected regions on the East Coast, you need to be *especially careful* about your drinking water.

Scientific American reports that after the hurricane, "several wastewater treatment plants [went] offline in New Jersey, and raw sewage carrying high levels of bacteria and viruses emptied into some waterways in the northern part of the state. Scientists estimate millions of gallons of sewage were spewed into New Jersey's rivers, streams and estuaries."[8]

Remember, it doesn't take an event on the scale of Hurricane Sandy to pollute your water with sewage. Each year, rainstorms across the country will make sewers overflow and potentially contaminate the tap water we drink.

Regulating Our Water: What's Allowed?

We've seen the effects of industrial and nonpoint source pollution, and the dangers of flooding and sewage overflow and some of the potential health effects they can have. But how much of that pollution actually makes it into our tap water? For the answer to that, let's take a quick look at the law that regulates your tap water.

Two years after the passage of the Clean Water Act, the Safe Drinking Water Act (SDWA) of 1974 was established to regulate the quality of our country's water supply and protect public health. SDWA has helped the United States come a long way in regulating some of the most harmful contaminants.

But right now the Safe Drinking Water Act regulates only about ninety chemicals and does not *prohibit* the presence of these toxic chemicals in our drinking water. Instead, it sets "safe" standards for chemicals such as cyanide, uranium, mercury, and lead. This means that each day, if you drink your municipal tap water, you are potentially ingesting these chemicals. On the EPA website, you can see a list of the contaminants allowed in our tap water.[9] Over the long term, these chemicals build up in our system and contribute to our overall toxic load, stressing the immune system and lowering our ability to handle allergens. Many toxins themselves also trigger allergic reactions.

Let's think about a rain barrel for a moment. As it fills up with water to the brim, it will soon overflow. This is the same thing that happens to your body. Your body has only so much room to carry that toxic load. Soon it will be overflowing with symptoms, and it becomes harder to fight off illness and allergies. The key here is to reduce our exposure and accumulation of toxins.

Unregulated Contaminants

Arsenic, cyanide, and uranium are among the approximately ninety chemicals the Safe Drinking Water Act regulates; however, there are over *sixty thousand* others used in industrial processes and other human activities that the SDWA *does not* cover. Since 2000, not one new chemical has been added to the list of regulated toxins. Yet new chemicals are added to our hygiene products, cars, paints, and electronic gadgets every day.

If you want to get your water tested for these and other chemicals, call the Safe Drinking Water Hotline (800-426-4791) provided by the EPA, or call any certified lab that can evaluate your drinking water. The phone numbers to these labs are available at your local EPA office or on its website.

THE FLUORIDE CONTROVERSY

When it comes to our tap water, perhaps no chemical generates such strong and wide-ranging opinions as fluoride.

Fluoride is a compound produced from fluorine, one of the naturally occurring elements, and is found in many products we use every day. Toothpaste and mouth rinses are well known for containing fluoride. Much of our food and beverages are packaged; therefore, if fluoridated water is used during the manufacturing process, your intake of fluoride may be much higher than you think or than is recommended. Fluoride is found in most packaged fruit juices, sodas, soups, coffee, and green and black tea; in prescriptions such as antibiotics, anesthesia, and fluoride supplements; and in insecticides and cleaning agents.

The United States and Canada started adding fluoride (fluorosilicic acid, sodium silicofluoride, and sodium fluoride) to the public water supply during the 1940s, after the U.S. Public Health Service recommended fluoride in public water supplies to help prevent dental caries (tooth decay). Concentrations were set at about one part fluoride per million parts water. According to the National Institutes of Health, about two-thirds of the U.S. population receives fluoride through community water systems. And yet the International Society for Fluoride Research, using data from the World Health Organization, finds that since 1965 tooth decay has declined in eight fluoridating countries (Australia, Canada, Hong Kong, Iceland, Israel, New Zealand, Singapore, and the United States) *and* in eight *nonfluoridating* countries (Japan, the Netherlands, Norway, Portugal, Spain, Sweden, Switzerland, and the UK).[10] This leaves the role of fluoride in preventing tooth decay murky at best.

Pure water is an *essential* nutrient—the basis of all living organisms and necessary to sustain life. To prevent disease, we need water that is clean and free of toxins and microbes. In adding fluoride to our drinking water, we are treating it as an oral medication to prevent a specific physical disease: dental caries, or tooth decay. But no disease has ever been linked to a fluoride deficiency.

> Pure water is an *essential* nutrient.

The more I researched, the more I was convinced that not only does *ingesting* fluoride provide no demonstrable benefit for the teeth but it has numerous harmful effects on the human body, such as skin irritation and respiratory issues. In addition, it increases our overall toxic load, contributing to more allergic sensitivities.

In fact, about three million Americans are believed to have fluoride sensitivities that can cause allergic reactions. Many people also develop gastrointestinal issues from fluoride consumption, making them more sensitive to foods that might not otherwise trigger allergic symptoms. Others can develop eczema or dermatitis. Fluoride may also interfere with thyroid functioning, wearing the body down. Its contribution to our overall toxic load means headaches, joint pain, insomnia, and fatigue.

Besides these allergic symptoms, fluoride can produce dental or enamel fluorosis. In its milder form, dental fluorosis is a permanent discoloration of the tooth enamel with white mottled specks or white streaks. In its more severe forms, the teeth are left with unsightly brown marks. Dental fluorosis comes from *drinking* an excess of fluoride during childhood, usually from the first year of life to about eight years. The Centers for Disease Control and Prevention (CDC) website published a 2005 report showing that about 40 percent of U.S. adolescents suffer from some form of dental fluorosis.[11]

Of more concern, however, is *skeletal* fluorosis, a process similar to dental fluorosis that affects the entire body if extremely high quantities of fluoride are ingested. People with skeletal fluorosis experience joint pain and arthritic symptoms, osteoporosis, and in more severe cases, skeletal deformation, limited range of motion, and crippled bones. While India and China are the two nations with the most cases of skeletal fluorosis, UNICEF claims that "fluorosis is endemic in at least 25 countries across the globe."[12]

Finally, fluoride may also have a link to cancer. In 2001, Paul

My Fluoride Story

My father worked for the U.S. Army in Seoul, Korea, and I was born at the Eighth Army U.S. Hospital on the Yongsan Military Base. I was one of the few Korean children lucky enough to attend the U.S. military school. Most of my friends were army brats, and every two years, I would have to make a fresh new group of friends. As long as I can remember, we had yearly "fluoride treatment day," when all the children gathered in the cafeteria to chew on red pills that would show if we had excess plaque, and then the teachers would force us to brush our teeth for ten minutes with heavily fluoride-medicated toothpaste. It tasted disgusting, and I just wished I were brave enough to skip school that day! Little did I know that the fluoride toothpaste was harmful to my body. Fast-forward to today. One of the main reasons I am such a strong proponent of living fluoride free is because, after many years of insomnia, I finally figured out that one of the major reasons for my sleeplessness was my exposure to, and accumulation of, fluoride during my childhood and adult years. Over the years, I ingested plenty of toxic fluoride antibiotics (for childhood throat infections), fluoridated tap water, foods containing high levels of fluoride, and plenty of matcha green tea. (Tea plants absorb fluoride from the soil.) Once I eliminated the hidden fluoride exposure, the high levels of fluoride in my urine decreased and soon my sleepless nights transformed to deeper uninterrupted sleep. I believe sleep is one of the most important health basics for longevity, which is why I call it one of the secrets to the fountain of youth.

Connett, professor of chemistry at St. Lawrence University, released a document titled "50 Reasons to Oppose Fluoridation." Among the reasons he cites for banning fluoride in our tap water are the carcinogenic effects observed in laboratory studies of rats, and two epidemiological studies showing a higher incidence of cancer in young men living in fluoridated areas.[13]

Given all these reasons to be leery of fluoridation, many communities have removed it entirely from their drinking water. Los Altos Hills, California; Boca Raton, Florida; San Antonio, Texas; Billings, Montana; and Lake Tahoe, Nevada, are among the dozens of cities that do not use it because of its potential adverse health effects.[14]

Despite all the problems of water pollution and the widespread use of fluoridation, I'm optimistic. I do believe that it's vitally important to address our environmental problems and search for realistic long-term solutions. Every act we take to improve the state of our earth will someday mean cleaner water for us, our children, and future generations to drink. Cleaner water going into our bodies means better allergy-reducing potentials.

WATER IN OUR BODIES: THE UNIVERSAL SOLVENT

So what does water do in our bodies? And how can it help you eliminate allergy symptoms?

Water is crucial for our survival and for the functioning of all our intricately connected bodily systems. The flow of blood, the lymphatic system, endocrine secretion, cellular detoxification, the urinary system, perspiration, saliva, tears, sexual secretions, lactation—all these natural bodily fluids depend on water. Getting important hormones and white blood cells to where they need to be depends on water. Our moods and feelings, the clarity of our thoughts—all these depend on water.

In working with allergies, water's power to act as a solvent is vital. The better hydrated you are, the more you dilute the concentration of allergens and toxins, reducing their potency and minimizing their harmful effects. Water can then flush the allergens out by increasing lymphatic activity and detoxifying them by way of the liver and kidneys, so they can be excreted through urination and bowel movements.

One of my favorite books on water is Dr. Fereydoon Batmanghelidj's *Your Body's Many Cries for Water.* He states that when the body is dehydrated, it naturally reacts by increasing histamine production. Histamine is one of many chemicals released by the immune cells (mast cells) during an allergic reaction. Histamine causes runny nose, runny eyes, hives, lung congestion, itching, and so on.

Batmanghelidj also believes that histamine is an important chemical for regulating our thirst mechanism, prompting us to increase our water intake, which flushes out allergens from our system, and to preserve water for vital physiological functions. We are all too familiar with over-the-counter drugs that mask the symptoms of allergies. They are mostly known as antihistamines. Antihistamines stop our immune system from producing histamines, muting the body's natural call for water during allergy attacks and, ultimately, causing dehydration of the cells. By using these drugs, we are countering our body's ability to flush out toxins. We are stopping the flow of water to heal the body.

All Dried Up

Marcus came to my office with severe asthma and chronic rhinitis. He brought in a large binder filled with medical reports from his pediatrician, allergist, and pulmonologist and from his many hospitalizations. He was only six years old, and for most of his young life, he had suffered from breathing problems.

All year long, he had nasal congestion, runny nose, and fatigue. Every other month, he would have severe asthmatic reactions that lasted for a week, when he needed breathing treatments with prescription drugs to open up his airways and reduce the inflammation.

His physical examination had telltale signs of dehydration: His skin was dry, flaky, and even wrinkled in certain areas such as his abdomen and neck. When I asked him to stick out his tongue, it was very dry, thin, and had deep crevices indicative of dehydration. When I asked his mother how often he had a bowel movement, she said maybe two times a week (daily is normal). His urine was scant and very dark in color.

This child was clearly dehydrated. When I asked how much purified water he drank she said, "Not much water at all—just juice and milk."

Right then I took him to my reception area, where I had purified water available, and gave him a large cup. I then gave specific instructions to his mother to give Marcus six cups of water per day, sipped slowly throughout the day, and absolutely no juice or milk. Sugar dehydrates cells, and milk causes excess mucus production because of its allergenic properties. I also put him on my allergy makeover dietary protocol.

At their follow-up visit one week later, two things visibly stood out: Marcus was energetic and actually looked as though he had gained some weight—his face and body looked more plump just from being hydrated.

Both Marcus and his mother were delighted because he had slept through the past few nights without needing to blow his nose or waking up choking on his own phlegm. From increasing his water intake, his body was naturally healing his allergies at the cellular level and reducing his histamine output. And ultimately, after a couple of months of regular hydration and being on my allergy makeover program, Marcus was free of his asthmatic symptoms.

I was tremendously proud of Marcus for following my recommendations, because up until then he hadn't liked the taste of water. Now he loves it!

THE SOLUTION: 4 STEPS TO CLEAN UP YOUR WATER

You would think that by now our society would have understood just how important clean water is to our overall well-being. With all this evidence before us, I believe we have a clear choice: We can either keep using our tap water or make a small but significant life change.

Bottom line: There is no reason to keep using tap water. Neither cost nor convenience should stand in the way of your and your family's health. Doing everything you can to *minimize* your exposure to all harmful chemicals, including mercury, lead, fluoride, arsenic, and the thousands of other unregulated chemicals in your tap water, is not just practical, it's good for your health and for reducing allergy symptoms.

Let me show you how. I invite you to incorporate the following four steps into your lifestyle so you can safely remove toxins, particulate matter, and microbes from tap water and start using pure, clean water's natural healing properties to reduce the toxic load and allergy symptoms that are preventing you from living with joy, vitality, and strength.

Step 1: Drink Plenty of Water

The human body is 60 percent water. Blood is 92 percent water, our brain is 70 percent water, and our muscles are 75 percent water. That's a whole lot of water!

Americans often don't drink enough water. What's more, coffee, soda, alcohol—all these are dehydrating, to the point that you might need a glass or more of water just to make up for the dehydration these drinks cause. In fact, to fight those allergies successfully, most of us just need to be drinking *more* purified water.

1. CONSUME PURIFIED WATER. Today, take it upon yourself to begin drinking purified water. This will cut down on the harmful chemicals, heavy metals, natural elements, and allergens you have been drinking for years.

I recommend that you buy purified bottled water until you can install a reverse osmosis unit (see step 2).

While you already know about the dangers of tap water, the filtered water from your refrigerator and even some bottled waters are not necessarily better. When you do buy bottled water, make sure the label on the bottle says that the water has been filtered and processed through a reverse osmosis (RO) filter. I prefer a triple filtration process in which the water bottler also ozonates the water to kill all microbes and uses a carbon filter system.

If it's available in your area, buy water in glass bottles rather than plastic. As we will see in later chapters, plastics should be avoided, especially when it comes to the foods you eat and the water you drink. You may also order your water monthly from a company if you prefer, but make sure it's reverse osmosis filtered water, and not spring or fluoridated water.

While buying bottled water is not a cost-effective long-term solution, it is a first step you can do *today* to get you on the right track to reducing allergies.

2. DRINK THE RIGHT AMOUNT OF PURIFIED WATER. By properly filtering your water, you'll stop ingesting allergens, microbes, and chemicals *from* the water. But as we talked about, most Americans don't drink *enough* water.

Only by getting enough water do you really let it do its allergy-reducing work in your bloodstream. You'd be surprised how many of my patients feel more alert and awake just by properly hydrating. Being dehydrated is like having a hangover without even knowing it. Worse still, dehydration slows us down and slows down our body's healing ability, exacerbating our allergic symptoms.

> Most Americans don't drink enough water.

Still, the right amount of water to drink is not the same for every person. Alas, the rule most of us have heard of "eight eight-ounce glasses" (sixty-four ounces) may not apply to you. The proper amount of purified water all depends on your weight.

> **Dr. Bennett's law for optimal water consumption for allergies:** Drink one-half of your body weight (pounds) in ounces of purified water every day. For example, if you weigh 160 pounds, you should drink 80 ounces of water. If you also drink caffeinated beverages, soda, or alcohol, the amount of water you need may be even higher.

But did you know that *how* you drink your purified water is also important? It's important not to "guzzle" water, or you'll lose its hydrating benefits. Just think of watering a small plant with a garden hose. Most of the water will either splash out or pour out the bottom. But if you water it with a slow trickle, the dirt absorbs the water to nourish the plant. Your cells are the same way: when you drink water slowly you give your cells time to absorb the water. Also, keep in mind that room-temperature water is easier on the digestive system than cold or ice water. Sipping water will also reduce the frequency of urination because it takes longer for the water to pass through your system.

If you or your child is athletic and sweats regularly, you'll need to drink more purified water. And if you live at high altitude or in the desert, where there is less moisture in the air, you need more water. Also, be mindful of adding more water to your daily intake during summer months.

Drink most of your purified water between meals, not during your meals. We want you to have the highest concentration of digestive enzymes to break down your food for proper assimilation. Drinking a lot of water during your meals dilutes the concentration of enzymes, affecting your ability to digest and assimilate important nutrients.

Action item. Calculate the amount of water your body needs (half your weight in pounds, then convert to ounces). Buy purified water, and sip it slowly at room temperature. Add more purified water to your daily intake if you live in drier climates, during the summer months, and if you are exercising.

Step 2: Buy a Reverse Osmosis Filtration Unit

OK, if you're ready to jump straight to the long-term water solution, here's how.

Buy a reverse osmosis (RO) filtration unit for installation at your kitchen sink. Most units are attached under the counter, with a spout up above going into the sink, so you may need someone who is handy to help you. Bottled water is a good first step, but the plastic, which is a known allergen, can leach into the drinking water and get absorbed in the body. Likewise, many companies bottle their water from mountain springs, which often flow through granite—which can have minute levels of uranium or arsenic.

In southern California, most of our water originates from the Colorado River. Granite rock, which contains uranium and arsenic, makes up much of the Rocky Mountains. Although these are naturally occurring geological contaminants, ingesting them in high amounts can be detrimental to the human body and can trigger allergic symptoms and irritations. Spring water sounds refreshing, but be cautious and, most important, be informed.

Reverse osmosis units will filter out these heavy metals, along with other natural and synthetic toxins, microbes, debris, and minerals. RO water is as pure as it gets, 100 percent H_2O.

With RO water there is only one drawback: depending on the unit, the wastewater (water that is poured down the drain while making purified water) can be high.

IS RO WATER "DEAD" WATER? Many patients challenge me with this question, protesting, "There are no minerals in RO water!"

Yes, both distilled water and reverse osmosis water are devoid of minerals, but ingesting mineral-free purified water is *not* harmful to your body. Did you know that rainwater is distilled water? People in most developing countries still drink rainwater. It is pure H_2O. Minerals such as calcium, magnesium, potassium, and sodium are absolutely essential to our cellular metabolism, growth and development, and general vitality. But we get most of our minerals from *eating food*, not drinking water. Eat plenty of vegetables, fruits, nuts, and seeds, and you will be optimally mineralized as well as balanced in alkalinity.

If you are overly concerned about the lack of minerals in RO water, you can remineralize each glass with a tiny pinch of Dead Sea salt. (You should not be able to taste the salt.) You may ask, why Dead Sea salt? It's because Dead Sea salt has a much lower sodium content (only 8 percent) and higher levels of calcium, magnesium, potassium, and sulfates than other salts, such as Himalayan salt, which has 98 percent sodium content. If Dead Sea salt isn't available, you can use regular sea salt—again not enough to taste.

Water bottling companies usually use a triple purification system: carbon filtration (removes chlorine, other chemicals, and larger particulates), ozonation (eradicates microbes), and reverse osmosis (removes heavy metals, aluminum, and nuclear material.) You can buy purified drinking water in large bottles (preferably glass) from delivery service companies and water service stores and clubs.

HOW DO RO FILTERS WORK? Reverse osmosis units work by pushing all your tap water through a semipermeable membrane, which collects the chemicals and bacteria and other microbes. The water passes through, and the bad guys are trapped. This filtration eliminates particles less than one-thousandth the diameter of a human hair, even down to the tiniest bacteria and parasites.

After membrane filtration, the unit should send the water through a carbon filter to remove gases and the bad tastes and odors in your tap. For this reason, when you buy your reverse osmosis unit, make sure it also has carbon filtration.

While still not perfect, reverse osmosis filtration can eliminate 95 percent or more of the harmful chemicals from your water. That allows your body to focus on other allergy culprits you may have—

pollen, fungi, dust mites—instead of on toxic chemicals in your tap water. I'll take 95 percent effective any day.

If you can't afford to buy an RO unit immediately (most models sell for under $200), buy purified water from the grocery store or order from a delivery service (glass bottles if possible) until you can. Each week, put aside as much money as you can toward a reverse osmosis fund. Think of it as an antiallergy savings plan!

Although I would rather have natural spring water because of its higher mineral content, I choose to have purified water because I know for sure that all the toxins have been removed by the reverse osmosis method. Spring water is not filtered by the RO process—it goes only through a carbon filtration system, which doesn't eliminate heavy metals and nuclear material.

Check your spring water source by calling the water bottling company and asking for the list of natural mineral content. You'll be surprised at the various minerals in bottled spring water— natural substances that are not known to be of value to the human body. And if your water comes from a well, definitely consider getting it analyzed. There are reputable water analysis laboratories that can help detect toxic metals and chemicals.

Action item. Go online and research RO units, then order one.

Step 3: Consider Buying a Whole-House Purification System

If you've already bought the reverse osmosis unit, you've taken a huge stride toward purifying the water you and your family ingest, and toward healing your allergy symptoms. Congratulations!

But let's not forget, ingestion isn't the only way water gets into our body. The skin absorbs water every time you wash your hands or take a shower. In the same way that a nicotine patch transfers chemicals into your bloodstream, every shower you take can do the same because the water we use in our home harbors chemicals that can produce allergies. Our cells are not like solid walls; they are porous and let in chemical messengers from the outside. And if your shower water is not filtered, the same chemicals that are in your drinking water can get absorbed through your skin.

To reduce your exposure to chemicals, heavy metals, chlorine, and microbes, I recommend getting a whole-house purification system. It will filter your water at the source. Every sink and shower in your home will flow with clean, fresh water, minimizing your exposure to waterborne allergens. Remember, this water, unlike RO water, is not for drinking. A whole-house filter is mainly a carbon filtration system.

Many people are sensitive to the chlorine that comes through showers and bathing, and a whole-house purification system is a great way to reduce your exposure. After all, a fifteen-minute shower means fifteen minutes of chlorine exposure that can cause headaches, itchy red eyes, runny nose, and skin irritations.

Whole-house purifiers are expensive, though; there's no getting around it. If you can't buy one right away, start a savings fund, each month putting away money toward the system. But start with your drinking water before moving on to the whole-house purification. What you drink always comes first.

Even if you don't have a whole-house purification system in place, there are some short-term fixes to help clean up your water.

If you live in a rental home or can't buy the whole-house purifier, start by buying a shower filter and attaching it to your showerhead. Don't waste your money on a little round filter (around $40); it will likely be clogged in a week. The type I recommend is about a foot long and is attached with an extension to the showerhead. Just about anyone can install it. These solid carbon block filters will eliminate chlorine, chemicals, and allergens from the water and usually cost from $125 to $150. I recommend changing the filter twice a year. You can also attach a shower hose at the end of the filter so that you can take a bath with clean water.

Action item. Research a whole-house filtration system online or immediately get an attachable shower filtration system and order a whole-house filtration system as soon as you can.

Step 4: Consider a Fluoride Filtration System

Now that we've eliminated most of the worst chemicals from your water, it's time to tackle fluoride. Shower filters and even whole-house filtration systems do not remove fluoride, even though it is a potential allergen.

The good news is, if your city doesn't fluoridate your municipal water, you are very lucky and you can skip this step. Call your city's department of water today and find out.

As we saw earlier, fluoride is not just in tap water but it can be found in foods, fruit juices, soda, soup, medication—almost anything that is manufactured with water.

As a result of all these inputs, your overall intake of fluoride may be much higher than you think—perhaps far exceeding safe, recommended amounts.

Even if you avoid fluoridated drinking water from your tap, you may be taking in more than you know when you shower, bathe, or even wash your hands. So in addition to your whole-house purification (which doesn't filter out fluoride), consider adding a fluoride filtration system.

Fluoride filters typically will use bone char, which is the most effective way of removing fluoride. Bone char consists of animal bones, which are high in calcium, heated to extremely high temperatures to optimize the ability to absorb and bind to fluoride.

Action item. Call your local department of water and find out if the city fluoridates the municipal water. If your city fluoridates your tap water, research fluoride filtration systems online and consider purchasing one.

I hope it's soaked in just how important water is to your body, and what cleaning it up can do to relieve your allergy symptoms. Pure water reduces the release of histamines and dilutes the concentration of toxins. Between neutralizing allergens and cleansing them out, keeping your blood and lymphatic systems going, and keeping your cells hydrated, water plays a crucial part in this seven-day process.

Now that we've focused on your food and water, we've eliminated some of the most proximate allergens you are likely to absorb. Simply by cutting down on these hidden allergy triggers, I expect that you will begin to feel better and facilitate your body's innate ability to heal.

DAY 3

CLEAN UP YOUR
AIR

Every day, trillions of plants around the world grow, photosynthesize, and release oxygen as part of their natural life cycle. The heating and cooling of oceans and earth, the formation of clouds, the precipitation of rain and snow—all these natural processes move air, and the oxygen in it, across the land. Incomprehensibly large numbers of oxygen atoms traverse the deserts, tundras, swamps, forests, and cities, yet only a minuscule fraction of them find their way into a living organism.

And every single day, one of those organisms is you.

Even without your control, your lungs expand and contract an average of twelve to eighteen times each minute, moving air into and out of your body. Sticky layers of mucus in your nose filter out bacteria, dust, and, yes, allergens that would otherwise make their way into your lungs and, ultimately, your bloodstream. You swallow this mucus, and your body naturally rids itself of countless allergens in your stomach and intestines.

The air makes it through your nose, then travels down your windpipe and into the alveoli, the tiny air sacs of your lungs, which bring oxygen into your bloodstream. Hitched to red blood cells, oxygen travels through the arteries and eventually converts the stored energy in the food you've eaten into high-potency chemicals to help all cellular processes—from the synaptic connections that produce a line of poetry to the muscle movements that make a toe wiggle. In exchange, carbon dioxide flows out of your alveoli, up through your windpipe, and back into nature. The planetary cycles of winds carry some small bit of this carbon dioxide (CO_2) to some of the trillions upon trillions of plants that make life possible for countless species of animals, including us. These plants thrive on the CO_2 we exhale. Using it in photosynthesis, they grow larger, reproduce, and prepare for the next cycle of plants that will produce the oxygen we breathe to survive.

As with our water supply, the condition of our air depends directly on the condition of the planet. Carbon monoxide, smog, car exhaust, pollution from heavy industry—all these things contribute to the graying of our planet's air and the graying of our lungs. Even a beautiful green spring meadow puts out pollens in the air, creating a blanket of yellow on our cars and outdoor furniture.

Unlike our food and water, air comes into our bodies unbidden. So while we can choose that high-powered salad over a bag of chips, or pure, reverse osmosis filtered water over municipal tap water, choosing to breathe in only the "best" air isn't so easy. Unless you are in an oxygen café, you inhale whatever is floating around in the environment. Pollen, dust, fungi, bacteria, toxic gases, and harmful chemicals will be in the air every day of our lives. But we can clean up our environment and strengthen our body's immunity, reducing allergy symptoms naturally.

If you've already implemented the protocols from Day 1 and Day 2, I'm hoping that you are now experiencing some positive changes in your body, indicating that your symptoms are abating. Remember, the body is an integrated whole, not a mere collection of subsystems. That means purifying your water and eating allergen-free foods will go a long way to help your body deal with allergens, whether they come by land, sea, or air!

The best solution is to avoid what we can and take extra care to create an allergen-free environment inside and outside the body. This chapter gives you some practical, cost-effective ways to reduce your intake of harmful allergens, toxins, and microorganisms and to help you clean and refresh the air you breathe, creating a more healthful living space.

First, let's understand exactly what is in the air you breathe. That way, you know what to be on the lookout for.

AIRBORNE ALLERGENS AND TOXINS

Pollen

Millions of people around the world suffer from what is commonly known as hay fever. More patients come to me to find relief from pollen allergies (or what they *think* are pollen allergies) than for anything else. Symptoms include sneezing and runny nose; itchy, watery eyes; and sinus pressure and congestion. Patients complain that they have difficulty sleeping, are constantly fatigued, can't get their work done, and are miserable much of the time because life just isn't fun anymore. They have a hard time even going outside or summoning up the energy to live fully.

The number of over-the-counter drugs available for allergies is overwhelming. In the drugstore or supermarket shelves, you'll find whole rows of bottles and boxes. Before starting my allergy makeover program, many patients come into my office with bags of prescription drugs and medications to relieve their symptoms. And when the drugs work, people do experience a whole new world. They suddenly feel refreshed, awake, and alive. They can *breathe* again, and everything feels light and lovely . . . for a time.

Drugs can be miraculous because they mask the allergy symptoms. They *alleviate* the problem without eliminating it. Soon enough, the medication wears off or maybe it stops working. The itchy eyes come back, the sneezing starts up, and unwanted side effects can even set in. And before long, we're back at square one. And so, in recent years, more and more people have seen the value of all-natural remedies. They want a solution that doesn't involve more synthetic chemicals or more bandages slapped on a deep physical issue.

While pharmaceutical companies make millions of dollars every year on medications that treat the symptoms, they have never offered a drug that can get to the root of pollen allergies. Allergy drugs are all about reducing or eliminating the symptom, never about the cure. The good news is that you are not doomed to a life of pollen allergies. Instead of taking more drugs, getting to the root means looking at your whole lifestyle and surroundings. That's how you discover why your body is sensitive to pollen in the first place. Why does pollen trigger symptoms in you but not in other people? What is going on in your body that makes it harder to eliminate the pollen buildup? Why is your immune system sensitive to these chemicals but not those?

> Allergy drugs are all about reducing or eliminating the symptom, never about the cure.

So just what does pollen do? Pollen is made of the male reproductive cells of plants; they float through the air during certain seasons (often spring). These cells land on plants perhaps dozens of miles away, find a mate, and, just as in human life, settle down and reproduce. This form of reproduction allows plants to create a great deal of genetic diversity over vast distances. So while it may cause you allergies, this mode of dissemination is actually part of the natural cycle of plant life.

Unfortunately, that doesn't make your symptoms any better.

A common misconception is that when it comes to pollen, flowers are worse than grass and trees. Not true. Bright, flowering plants are usually pollinated by bees or other animals. Because pollen from flowers hitches a ride on the legs or wings of bees, butterflies, birds, and even bats, it doesn't need to float through the air. And whatever these creatures carry off on their feet and wings isn't likely to end up in your nasal passages. Most of the pollen that bothers us comes from ragweed; coniferous trees; broadleaf trees such as oak, elm, and birch; herbaceous plants such as sagebrush and tumbleweed; and all kinds of grasses, such as bluegrass, Bermuda grass, and the countless varieties found in suburban lawns.

If you have a pollen allergy, you'll probably know it, because symptoms will ebb and flow with the seasons, depending on where you live. It's often worst in the morning, when pollen counts are high. The website Pollen.com has a helpful color-coded graph that tells you how much pollen is in the air in your region. Be especially careful on high-pollen, red alert days.

Many people also confuse common cold symptoms with pollen allergies (hay fever). Hay fever may feel like a cold at first, but you won't get a fever. Colds tend to go away fairly quickly—say, in under a week—whereas pollen allergies linger often for weeks or months. Likewise, longer-term allergy symptoms (that go beyond a single allergy season) are probably caused by something in your home. Many people think they have pollen allergies when, in fact, the real culprit is dust mites or mold. We'll cover what to do about those in the next chapter.

There's a good chance that if you're reading this book, you are worried about pollen allergies. That's because, at any given time, one in ten people in the United States has pollen allergies, with some estimates putting that number higher. Anywhere from 30 to 40 percent of people will develop a pollen allergy at some point during their lifetime. In the second part of this chapter, you will learn how to keep pollen out of your home and how to clean up the pollen that does get in. Don't forget, pollen settles on your hair and clothes, and even if you don't inhale these particles at first, they can be transferred to your pillows and sheets, where you almost certainly will contact and inhale them. Your cleaning ritual will also become part of your 7-Day Allergy Makeover, and you'll learn when to open and shut your windows, how you circulate the air in your car. By implementing simple and practical tips to reduce your pollen allergies, you will be breathing better, and have more energy, in no time.

Pollution and Toxins

Pollen may be irritating, but it's not toxic. That doesn't make the suffering any easier to deal with, but it's good to know it isn't causing cancer or damaging your lungs. Some of the chemicals we're about to look at—ones you breathe *every day*—not only produce a whole range of allergenic effects such as headaches, watery eyes, rashes, brain fog, and lethargy but also damage the functioning of your bodily systems. Carbon monoxide and smog are well known, but sulfur dioxide, nitrogen oxides, and volatile organic compounds (VOCs) are also cause for concern.

Most of the chemicals we're going to learn about come directly from human sources. They are the result of heavy industry, car exhaust, wood and coal burning, plastics, and paints, to name a few. In the course of a year, some ten billion tons of toxic chemicals are added to the global air supply. If only the tiniest fraction of those pollutants makes its way into your lungs, you're likely to feel the effects. Not only are you going to feel the allergic symptoms but you will also be increasing your toxic load, disrupting the cellular metabolic function of your tissues, and harming your ability to handle other allergens.

The emissions we hear about most in the news is carbon dioxide. While not an allergen, CO_2 is the major contributor to the global carbon footprint and, quite likely, the global upswing in droughts, hurricanes, and floods that has marked the past few years. Increasing CO_2 emissions can sometimes also indicate an upswing in emissions of the other toxic chemicals we're going to discuss a little later. The truth is, cars, airplanes, factories, and other polluters emit a host of gases harmful to human beings, including carbon monoxide, sulfur dioxide, nitrogen oxides, and particulate matter. These chemicals, along with lead and ozone, are currently regulated under the Clean Air Act (roughly the equivalent of the Safe Drinking Water Act and the Clean Water Act, but for air). International standards for greenhouse gas reduction remain a critical issue for helping slow down climate change and making the air friendlier to those with allergies. Chemicals from Mexico can drift to Los Angeles, and vice versa. Here the local truly is the global.

With this reality in mind, more than 190 countries have become signatories to the now-famous Kyoto Protocol, which set benchmarks for the reduction of greenhouse gases, including CO_2, usually at or near the 1990 year levels. Yet only a fraction of those countries—mostly those in the European Union—actually established tangible and binding targets for greenhouse gas reduction. Although the United States, has never ratified the Kyoto Protocol, it became the first major industrial nation in the world to meet the targeted reductions of carbon dioxide emissions required in 2012.

However, since the time of the Kyoto Protocol, we have seen the emergence of large new economies in China, India, Brazil, and elsewhere. These countries, experiencing huge economic growth while polluting the environment at ever-expanding rates, feel limited responsibility for the devastation they are creating. One of the challenges going forward will be not only to get the United States to reduce its emissions but also to find a way to encourage these rapidly developing countries to comply with international environmental standards without stifling their growth.

Even though we're breathing cleaner air than we were forty years ago, these chemicals still pose serious problems for anyone suffering from allergies and respiratory illnesses. Let's take a look at some of the pollutants that you may be inhaling today.

SULFUR OXIDES. Remember acid rain? It created quite a big scare back in the 1980s but seems to have disappeared from our news. While tougher regulations are in place to help clean it up, the problem of acid rain hasn't gone away. Happily, it is no longer melting marble statues and antiquities at an alarming rate, but it still pollutes the environment and harms our health. Sulfur oxides and nitrogen oxides are the two main culprits in acid rain.

At the larger, environmental level, acid rain causes water sources on the ground to become more acidic, endangering aquatic and marine life and vegetation. And, of course, acid rain is harmful to humans, too. It doesn't burn your skin or smell like a sulfur pit. In fact, it doesn't look or feel or taste any different from normal rain. But this type of rain (and acid snow, mist, and fog too) increases your chances of inhaling or otherwise ingesting the harmful compounds that have mixed into the water.

But a more likely allergy concern than acid rain is the sulfur dioxide you inhale as it enters the atmosphere and travels out of the industrial areas in your region.

Sulfur dioxide (SO_2), is a chemical released from many industrial processes, especially from coal-burning power plants, which are a major source of smokestack pollution. It can provoke a wide variety of symptoms, including irritation of the skin and eyes. But its most notable consequences all have to do with the respiratory system. Sulfur dioxide is known for provoking asthmatic reactions, and it can create other breathing difficulties. According to the EPA, sulfur oxides (including SO_2) can cause emphysema and bronchitis, aggravate existing heart issues, leading to hospitalizations and premature death. Both animal and occupational studies confirm that it can inflame or even destroy parts of the lungs. It makes handling airborne allergens that much more difficult if your system is already trying to deal with sulfur dioxide.

Whether they come in acid rain or in the air we breathe, we need to minimize our exposure to sulfur dioxide.

NITROGEN OXIDES. Like sulfur oxides, nitrogen oxides are released into the atmosphere by the burning of coal, oil, and gas. They are also released from kerosene heaters, wood-burning stoves, auto exhaust, and cigarette smoke (and, yes, that means it's in secondhand smoke). Along with their contribution to environmental degradation, nitrogen oxides have similar effects to those of sulfur dioxide, causing skin and throat irritations, shortness of breath and general difficulty in breathing, fatigue, and nausea. Nitrogen dioxide is also one of the main ingredients in that noxious mixture known as smog, which we will discuss further.

VOLATILE ORGANIC COMPOUNDS. VOCs are solvents such as formaldehyde, toluene, benzene, xylene, methylene chloride, and perchloroethylene. They are often found in paints, inks, glues, tobacco smoke, particleboard furniture, pesticides, building products, vinyl flooring, marking pens, and much more. They have an array of allergenic effects, including eye and throat irritation, headache, fatigue, rapid heartbeat, dizziness, joint pain, nausea, insomnia, and difficulty in concentrating. They are also suspected of being carcinogenic to humans (and are proven carcinogens to animals). At higher levels, they can even cause damage to the internal organs and nervous system.

A Raspy Voice Improves

Anyone who has ever heard my voice will tell you that it is definitely raspy and lower in tone than you might expect from someone with my small frame. But during chiropractic school, after learning about some of the causes of vocal strain, I got quite concerned. I went to a reputable doctor, who diagnosed me with vocal cord nodules. He prescribed speech lessons, but after six months, I quit because it never changed my tone or smoothed out the raspiness. My voice would get raspier at times, but if I just shut up, it would get better overnight. For years, that was the state of my voice.

Until I was on maternity leave. After spending six weeks out of the office, I noticed that my voice was clear, free of strain, and actually rather high in pitch. I just thought that maybe I had strained my voice from talking to my patients, but as soon as I went into my office for a day to get ready for my first week back—a day without any patients—my voice started cracking, and the raspiness came right back. Again, I wasn't talking to patients, I was simply at my office, cleaning up and organizing my files. This was a big clue!

I started to look around my office for chemicals and toxins that could be the root cause of my vocal strain. I looked all around: no glues, permanent marking pens, perfumes, or cleaning agents. Just particleboard, laminated office furniture, carpet, and vinyl furniture. So . . . what did all these have in common? VOCs!

I did more detective work and started to think back over all the years I had a strained voice, and sure enough, it all started when I moved to the States. In Korea, we never had carpeting, and all the floors were made of real wood. We didn't have any new furniture, only Korean antiques. And we slept on the floor with futon-style beds that were all silk and cotton.

After more research, it hit me. All the products in my office were outgassing formaldehyde, a VOC. I realized right then that my vocal nodules had developed from formaldehyde poisoning, from the ten years of dissection, starting in eighth grade and continuing all the way into chiropractic school! Ten years of breathing in the formaldehyde that preserved all my anatomical specimens: earthworms, frogs, fetal pigs, and human cadavers. Once the nodules formed, they just got exacerbated by being exposed to the cheap office furniture.

I also started noticing that every time I went into a shopping mall, my voice would get worse. I was just like the canary in the coal mine—my voice would tell me if I was around formaldehyde. Pretty cool to have my own warning system, but it definitely came at a price.

If you were to come into my office today, you would see that the office furniture is all wood. I have tile flooring, and my bookshelves and painted walls are VOC free. I even have a special type of air purifier that absorbs formaldehyde and other types of chemicals. My voice is much better than it used to be, but I think my nodules will be there for life.

Old paint cans lying around the garage (or, worse, in the house) emit VOCs, as do many cleaning products. Even clothes returned from the dry cleaner's may not be safe. VOCs are everywhere in our household products (even our shampoos); in the next chapter, you'll learn how to eliminate them from your home. Ambient VOCs, whether outgassed from paints and adhesives or released from factories, find their way into the atmosphere and build up with nitrogen oxides. Mix in a little sunlight, and you have that most famous of urban blights: photochemical smog.

GROUND-LEVEL OZONE (SMOG). Far from being simply a matter of smoke mixed with fog (as the original coiner of the term thought), smog is a noxious mixture of acidic chemicals, particles, and gases that damage your lungs, irritate your eyes, and make life a little more glum. Think of a rough urban neighborhood, and you'll probably think of smog. And as we know, smoggy days are especially brutal for allergy sufferers.

This mixture of sulfur and nitrogen oxides, sunlight, and volatile organic compounds reacts to produce particulate matter and ground-level ozone (O_3). Yes, the very ozone that protects us from harmful ultraviolet rays in the atmosphere is the same stuff that leads to such problems down here at ground level. This is one ozone layer we should seek to destroy!

An American Lung Association report, "State of the Air 2012," shows 41 percent of Americans live in places with high levels of industrial and automobile pollution. At the most basic level, the ozone in smog causes irritation or burning in the lungs and can lead to reduced lung function in general. And because ozone can trigger asthmatic reactions, asthma sufferers need to be especially aware of their surroundings on smoggy days.

But ozone has more serious long-term health effects. The EPA says that it may aggravate the effects of emphysema and chronic bronchitis and even "make the lungs more susceptible to infection."[1] Like so many other allergens, ozone doesn't just trigger immediate effects; it also wears your body down from its optimal state, making it difficult to deal with other respiratory allergens.

Further, the particulate matter that separates during the chemical reactions that produce smog generates problems of its own. "Particulate air pollution is consistently and independently related to the most serious effects, including lung cancer and other cardiopulmonary mortality."[2] That means it's not just sulfur dioxides and VOCs but soot, dust, sand, and other particles that get inhaled or ingested on especially smoggy days.

The reality is that most of us live in areas that are smoggy. Los Angeles, where I live, is certainly the unrivaled champion of smog generation in the United States. Because we can't avoid smog altogether, I'll show you some practical ways around it, whether you're at home, outdoors, or even stuck in traffic.

CARBON MONOXIDE. Carbon monoxide (CO) is one of the deadliest of the toxic gases, and it's found all around us. And while we've all heard horror stories about carbon monoxide–related deaths, it also can have some less serious but still harmful consequences for you and your allergies.

Emitted from smokestacks everywhere, carbon monoxide also comes out of our heaters, water heaters, ranges, furnaces, and fireplaces and spews out of our car exhaust pipes. With so many places in the home producing invisible carbon monoxide gas, this is one toxic chemical we need to be on a special lookout for. At lower levels, it can cause brain fog, headaches, lethargy, confusion, and difficulty concentrating. It also contributes to your toxic load, making it that much more difficult to handle other allergens. If you don't have a carbon monoxide detector already, please buy one and install it in your home. They're cheap, and if you can put a battery in a flashlight, you can install a detector. CO detectors will not warn you of smoke from fires (just a reminder to make sure your smoke detectors are also working!), but they will sound an alarm when carbon monoxide reaches a dangerous level, giving you time to vent your home and call for an inspection.

Unsafe practices can lead to carbon monoxide–related health issues. In the wake of Hurricane Sandy, thousands of people without electricity turned to generators to power their homes. And in New Jersey and Pennsylvania, several died from carbon monoxide poisoning because they were running generators indoors, which should *never* be done. Others have died from carbon monoxide inhalation after using camping stoves in confined spaces. Exhaust from idling cars and leaky furnaces has also claimed many lives. You must be knowledgeable and extremely cautious with any appliance that releases carbon monoxide.

CO Poisoning

My patient Misty is a young married woman with a four-year-old son and a six-year-old daughter. After a few nights in their newly built home, Misty's daughter woke her up in a panic. She complained of having a bad headache and not feeling well. But Misty quickly realized that she had a much bigger issue than her daughter: She couldn't *talk* to her daughter—she was slurring her speech and felt as if her face was paralyzed. Barely able to get up out of bed, she tried to walk but just fell to the floor. Although she was only thirty-three years old, she thought she was having a stroke.

She immediately woke up her husband, and they rushed to the nearest emergency room. The doctors found that her symptoms were not from a stroke but from dangerously high levels of carbon monoxide poisoning.

As soon as they mentioned CO poisoning, Misty felt a stab

of fear because her children and her parents were still in the house. She called them immediately to get out. How could this happen in a new house, and where could the CO be coming from? After all, their rooms were nowhere near the garage where their cars were stored.

They discovered that their contractor had installed a faulty pool heating unit that was adjacent to the master bedroom. Carbon monoxide was slowly being pumped into the house, through the master suite. Misty was very lucky. Her strokelike symptoms gradually dissipated, and she got back her energy and full use of her muscles. She did have some minor brain fog and memory issues, but I was able to help her restore her cognitive functions within a month of treatment. If not for her daughter and the fast action of the doctors, she might not be alive today.

A CDC bulletin reports that in 2001 and 2002, an average of 480 persons died annually from non-fire-related CO poisoning. Perhaps even more alarming, the study shows that another 15,200 people had to be treated in hospitals for nonfatal CO-related poisoning during 2001 to 2003. Problems with furnaces and heaters during the colder months were the largest contributing factor in these cases. These stories make us lament such easily preventable deaths. But these are only the stories that make the headlines.

People are harmed by carbon monoxide exposure every day. That's because carbon monoxide, in smaller quantities, may be roaming around your home right now without your knowing it. Even a little too much time in the garage after your car was left idling can do damage. Even the smallest CO leak in the house can be one of the major culprits in many allergy symptoms, including fatigue, brain fog, dizziness, headaches, and occasional nausea.

You may be surprised to know that it can also cause emotional issues. Panic, anxiety, and higher perceived stress levels are all reported by people who unwittingly inhale carbon monoxide. The lethargy caused by long-term exposure can even explain some cases of chronic fatigue. After many of my patients had their heating appliances checked, stopped using their fireplaces, and exercised more caution with car exhaust near doorways and windows, they felt much better and stronger. The brain fog lifted, and they felt sharp and alert again in a way they hadn't felt in years. Right now is a great time to get all the stoves and heating units in your house inspected and make sure they're functioning as they should. On your new quest to live allergy free, have an expert examine sources of carbon monoxide in your home and make sure everything is well sealed, well ventilated, and *safe*.

NEXT STEP?

Remember how we began the chapter talking about the great ecological cycles that bring oxygen into your body? Now that you've read about sulfur dioxide, ozone, particulates, pollen, and nitrogen oxides, you know that the air you're breathing is likely anything but pure.

When it comes to air pollution, your home is your first line of defense. Its walls, windows, floors, and roof block out what they can, providing a bulwark against these allergens. But inevitably, some of these harmful chemicals will get through. Pollen comes through the ducts or chimney. Sulfur dioxide sneaks in under the door. Particulate matter creeps through a window screen.

Your home should be the cleanest, most comfortable place for you to be. But if you have respiratory allergies, you know that your body feels as if it were being assaulted by the environment around you. For so many of my patients, the changes I am about to recommend have been real game changers. They have seen unbelievable turnarounds from the groggy, runny-nosed, sneezy allergy sufferers they thought they always would be, to the creatures brimming with life, light, and energy that I knew they were. With these tips, you will filter out the worst allergens and be better prepared to handle those that do make it into your home.

Combined with the tips in the next chapter, you'll make the air you breathe better than you could ever have imagined.

There are three basic tips for cleaning up your air, which are summarized as follows:

1. Block out what you can.
2. Filter everything else.
3. Don't add anything that makes allergies worse.

The first two are common sense. Closing doors and windows will do a lot of good, and proper filters and purifiers will take care of a lot of what they can't.

But the third tip will likely take some explaining.

With allergies, sometimes the cure can be worse than the symptom. Every year, people aggravate their allergies by using products that do more harm than good. If you have a cut, you don't squeeze lemon juice into it. In the same way, if you have an allergy problem, using products made of plastics, chemicals, and synthetics is not going to solve your issue in the long run. These will only add to the toxic buildup in your system and make your allergy problem worse. That's why, throughout the

> With allergies, sometimes the cure can be worse than the symptom.

book, I'm careful to delineate the types of products to buy (almost always organic, all natural, chemical free, made of things like iron, glass, and untreated wood), and those you should avoid (synthetic, processed, chemically treated).

AIR QUALITY IN YOUR HOME

While there is no way to keep our indoor air completely free of toxins, pollen, and other allergens, our homes are often unnecessarily *loaded* with them. In fact, our homes can be ten times more allergenic than the outdoors. Considering that most Americans spend about 90 percent of their time indoors, that's 90 percent of your life inhaling ten times the level of allergens you would if you were outside. That's why I can't stress it enough: after taking care of your food and water, *you must clean up your air.*

Step 1: Invest in an Air Purifier

Get an air purifier, and you will take care of up to 99 percent of airborne allergens in your home.

An air purifier is the most concentrated form of allergen-eliminating machinery you can find. A good one will clean and recirculate the air in your room two or three times an hour, eliminating most of the chemicals that are likely to leave you running for your handkerchief or wiping your eyes.

But not all air purifiers are created equal. Some are too small for your room. Others don't filter out everything you want them to. So how do you know what kind of purifier to get?

The magic word (or, in this case, acronym) is HEPA. For maximum effectiveness, get a HEPA air purifier with a carbon filtration system, all in a completely metal housing unit. Why metal? You avoid the outgassing of plastics and glues that hold the unit together.

HEPA stands for high-energy particulate air filtration. Do not settle for HEPA-type, HEPA-style, or HEPA-ish purifiers. Check and double-check the label. Knockoffs filter at significantly lower percentages and won't remove all the allergens you need to eliminate. Having a HEPA filter alone will do wonders. For one thing, it will eliminate particles down to 0.3 micrometers (aka microns). Consider that a human hair can be between 35 and 100 microns across; we're talking particles one-hundredth that size. This kind of filtering can eliminate a wide range of allergy triggers, such as pollen, dust mites, car exhaust particulates, and bacteria. Some filters can even get down to 0.1 micron (one ten-millionth of a meter).

Even so, filtering out these particles alone isn't enough. Your purifier should also have a carbon filtration system to eliminate the toxic gases we discussed earlier. A good carbon filter will capture volatile organic compounds and chemicals that are difficult to detect, such as formaldehyde, toluene, styrene, radon, natural gas, carbon monoxide, and perfumes. Some of these chemicals are known carcinogens, and all of them contribute to your toxic load. All are terrible for allergy sufferers.

Now, here is one final, crucially important aspect to the equation: you must make sure you have the *right type* of HEPA carbon-filtered air purifier. First, you want to measure your room size in square feet and buy the purifier that will optimally filter the air of your space. If your purifier is too weak, it won't circulate all the air, thus leaving you vulnerable to allergy attacks. And if the purifier is made of plastic, even though you are filtering the air, you are still introducing more plastic into your room, thus undermining your own efforts. Getting rid of some allergens by introducing others is not the way to go. (In the next chapter, we'll talk more about the case for eliminating, or at least reducing, *all* plastics.)

Step 2: Clean Your Air Ducts, Vents, and Filters

Air naturally travels through your home every day. How much of it comes through your ducts if you turn on your air-conditioning and heating unit? *A lot.* Let's make sure that the air flowing through the air ducts is as clean and clear of toxins as it can be. This will help reduce your nasal and sinus symptoms dramatically.

1. FILTERS. Air that makes its way through your ducts or vents will eventually run into a filter. These filters capture not just the chemicals and pollen we looked at in this chapter but also mold, dust, and other things too small to see. Air filter maintenance is not on top of every busy person's schedule.

Look at it this way, if you don't change your filters, you probably have months—make that *years*—of dust, mold, chemicals, and other allergens backed up in your ducts. Every time air blows through, it inevitably shakes loose some of those particles, forcing them into your home. You haven't really fixed the problem; you've just collected everything in one place. These inhalants will spread through the air, leading to upper respiratory issues (runny nose, congestion) and can even make you feel tired and irritable. Many people who believe they suffer from pollen allergies or hay fever may actually be suffering from a buildup of mold in their house's air ducts.

While standard protocol says to change your filters once a year, I recommend replacing them with every new season (four times a year) to keep your indoor air clean and free of particulates.

If you're not sure how to change the filters to your air-conditioner or home heating and cooling system, here are a few helpful tips:

- Identify the specific type and size of filter you will need for the heating or cooling unit. If you have your unit in the attic, you will also need one for the central return grill located in the ceiling.
- If your unit has a fresh-air intake, you will need to change the fresh-air filter, too.
- Go to your local hardware store with your old filter so you can get the right brand, and ask if they can recommend a better-quality filter. This is not the place to pinch pennies— those $1.99 filters won't do the job. Buy enough filters for the whole year.

2. AIR DUCTS. Now, even if your filters are clean, it doesn't mean that the ducts themselves are clean. Mold, dust, bugs, and the chemicals we've mentioned can get trapped in them and stay there for weeks or months. This is probably not a job for the faint of heart or anyone not inclined toward manual labor.

Get your air ducts cleaned at least once a year by a reputable company. And make sure they clean the complete duct system, not just around the air vents. Ask them not to use any chemicals such as fungicides or chemical cleaning agents. *Why?* The answer is simple: If those end up in your vents, you will be breathing them in for weeks. The air that passes into your home will pick up the chemicals, which can be just as bad as the molds and bacteria you were trying to get rid of in the first place. Keep the cleaning all natural so that what you breathe in will have the least impact on your respiratory system.

3. VENTS. Now that you've changed the filters and cleaned out the ducts, how clean are the vents in your house? These are the small grills on the walls or the floor where the heated or cooled air comes out, and the other ones where the room air goes back into the return ducts. They will need regular cleaning, too—about once a month! Wipe them down with a damp cloth. To clean off mold and debris, use a mixture of one part white vinegar and one part water.

4. WALL HEATERS. Many older apartments have wall heaters. I've seen dust piles on these I could hardly believe. Every time that hot air blows out, so does all that dust. To clean your wall heater, use a vacuum cleaner to suck out what you can from inside. Then simply take a wet paper towel to the outside to clean up the rest. Hard? No. But easy to forget about in the rush of a tough week? Of course. Make it part of your allergy makeover routine.

Step 3: Keep the Outside Air Out!

There is always a balance to strike between ventilating your home and keeping excess pollutants out. My rule of thumb is that whenever possible, close your windows to keep out airborne contaminants from your external environment.

Now, we all want a breath of fresh air, but what if inhaling smog, soot, and sulfur dioxide is the price you pay? The problem is, all these settle into your room and stay there, just waiting for you to inhale them. Every car that drives by is one more breath of exhaust. The brown haze of smog on the afternoon horizon is one more round of coughing or itchy eyes.

At night, mold and spores proliferate, making the world outside a fungal breeding ground. On windy days, pollen grains waft through the air, just waiting to make their way to your eyes, throat, and nose.

Another easy step—which is also a gracious gesture in many

cultures—is to leave your shoes at the door. It's amazing how many kinds of allergens such as pesticides, molds, and chemicals can just walk right into your house on the soles of your shoes. Try walking around in a pair of slippers or indoor shoes instead, and keep a basket of extras for guests.

If you live in high-fire zones, you absolutely must keep the windows closed during fire season because smoke and ash can make eyes itchy and cause breathing problems.

With your HEPA filtration unit, that air will feel better than ever. Keeping the windows shut is also a smart strategy for lowering the impact on your purifier.

Do open up your windows periodically, during calm and crisp mornings, to freshen up your house and move out stale air. *Then shut them.*

Step 4: Clean Up the Air in Your Car

You're zooming down the freeway at 8:00 a.m. You pass the businesswoman applying eyeliner, the session guitarist heading home after one too many hours at the recording studio, the sixteen-year-old with a terrified driving instructor. Life is good—no delays, no stalled cars on the freeway.

But on the commute, you notice something; your eyes are starting to itch. Your nose is sending that "something about to trickle out" message to your brain. Maybe a cough or two. And there they are again: allergies. Yes, allergens make it even this far, even into the confines of our precious automobiles. Can we *never* get away from them? Smog, particulate matter, car exhaust—by now, I'm sure you can imagine how bad these really are. And yet, when we drive they're all around us.

Because many of us spend eight to ten hours a week in our cars, this is a vitally important place to strike back against allergens.

Even with the windows rolled up, smog and exhaust can seep into the car and affect our breathing.

So, short of walking to work or riding a bike (which I encourage!), what can we do? Here are some simple changes that will help you minimize exposure to allergens while driving.

1. RECIRCULATE YOUR AIR. Before you start your engine, roll up your car windows and set your car to recirculate the air without letting outside air in. You can do this simply by pressing the "recirculate" button (normally indicated by a C-shaped arrow). This way, you'll have clean air during your drive in traffic. Avoid those toxic gases spewing out of the muffler of the car front of you.

And while you drive, be sure to keep your windows up.

2. GET RID OF CONTAMINANTS IN THE CAR. You know those green pine tree fresheners people hang on the rearview mirror? Would you be surprised to learn they are loaded with synthetic chemicals? Probably not. But what if I told you they can lead to brain fog and poor concentration?

For many people, these fresheners can cause allergic symptoms such as headache, wheezing, coughing, and congestion. Moreover, they can decrease your focus on the road, where it's all-important. So toss the fake tree. If you want your car to smell clean, here's a novel idea: just keep it clean! Which brings us to . . .

3. CLEAN UP THE CAR'S INTERIOR. As I just mentioned, the interior of your car, as well as your skin and clothes, can collect toxins and particulates anytime the windows are open. Some particulates might make it in even if the windows are closed. Washing the interior is one obvious way to remove these chemicals.

But wait—doesn't that local car wash place use harsh chemicals, too? It certainly can, and that's why you need to use an eco-friendly car wash. Patronize companies that offer all-natural, nontoxic car cleanings. Your car will smell better, and your nose won't feel the effects of fumes and chemicals. (Planet Earth will thank you too.)

4. KEEP THE CAR OUT OF THE GARAGE. In the old days, garages were meant for cars. Nowadays, they seem to be places to store the old basketball hoops, paint cans from the 1980s, six-foot-tall stacks of photo albums, and every stuffed animal you and your children ever had. Garages are often filled with our detritus, and this makes them a veritable cesspool for allergies.

You may not even park your car in the garage. And if you don't, my advice to you is to keep doing what you're doing! That's because, even if you miraculously do have enough space in the garage to fit your car, it's better to park it in the driveway or on the street. Sure, you risk a little rain, snow, or sleet, but your allergy load will decrease.

Exhaust and carbon monoxide from your car engine fills the garage every time you park. Worse, you may linger a minute, engine idling, and finish that song on the radio. Guess what? Even with the door open, more of that exhaust fills up the space. The song ends with a final guitar chord and drum roll, and you turn off the engine. You step out of your car, and . . .

There it is. Carbon monoxide. Exhaust. Particulate matter. You do this every Monday, Tuesday, Wednesday. . . . Your toxic load builds, and before you know it, you're vulnerable to all kinds of chemicals that weren't bothering you before.

But there's an even darker side to this story. Carbon monoxide from your garage can also drift into the house and even upstairs to second-floor bedrooms. If you have an attached garage, this no parking in the garage rule is especially vital. I've had patients who were accidentally exposing their families to these gases because of how close their garages were to their doors and windows.

5. BEWARE THAT NEW-CAR SMELL. Although most of us love

that new-car smell, it isn't on friendly terms with your allergies. Plastics and VOCs abound in new cars because such chemicals are often found in the paints, glues, and adhesives used in car manufacture.

If you buy a new car, here's how to make it an allergy-friendly one.

If it's brand new, roll down the windows a bit every night so that the VOCs can outgas. These chemicals, when inhaled in such a confined space, can cause a range of symptoms, including asthma, brain fog, confusion, anxiety, and lethargy. VOCs, remember, are part of the formula for making smog.

Buying a used car, even if it's only a year old, will save you this hassle because many of the chemicals will already have evaporated, and you will have saved almost half the price of a new car.

DAY 4

CLEAN UP YOUR
LIVING
ENVIRONMENT

THE HALFWAY POINT

Today is the halfway point in your seven-day journey. If you've made it this far, you're well on your way toward a new body and a new life. Overcoming allergies isn't easy. It means huge changes in your diet, your lifestyle, and the way you approach your health. So take a moment to reflect on how far you've come, and congratulate yourself. You've made some life-changing decisions.

Now, if you haven't implemented 100 percent (or even 10 percent) of the strategies I've recommended in the first three chapters, don't fret. Slowly work them into your life. Go back to the previous chapters and review what you've done and what you haven't. Take stock of what you still need to do to reach your goal of a new you. Let's say you've slacked on getting that water purifier. Maybe today you could simply look for one on the Internet. In a week, you could compare prices and call a few places to see what they have in stock. A week after that, who knows? You might buy one.

Now is a good time to fill out the allergy checklist again and compare it to how you felt before starting the 7-Day Allergy Makeover. Let's see just how different you feel and whether you can link the new you to some of the positive changes you made in your home and your diet. Your skin, digestive, and respiratory symptoms from food allergies can begin to recede after two to three days, and you may notice benefits from drinking purified water and breathing cleaner air. Once you finish filling out the checklist, look back over the one you filled out on Day 1. Notice how many symptoms you checked, and how you rated each one, the first time around. While we shouldn't expect them all to be gone after just three days, chances are good that you *are* feeling better than you were even a few days ago. Do you have more energy? Are you a little less congested and bloated? Do you feel less pressure in your sinuses? Are you feeling a bit lighter and freer in your body? Maybe even lost a few pounds? And, perhaps most important, how do you feel overall with the process of becoming allergy free? Are you jazzed and eager? Or frustrated and maybe a bit overwhelmed? Or maybe, at different times, all the above?

Be sure to keep track of your mental and emotional health as well, since these are essential to this transformative process. When it comes to allergies, slow and steady really does win the race. Make the changes you can, and always push yourself *just a little* outside your comfort zone. If you keep going, keep striving, and keep open to this process, I have no doubt that the results will speak for themselves.

CLEAN UP YOUR LIVING ENVIRONMENT

Today, we take a look at allergy-proofing your entire home (except for the kitchen, which we'll look at tomorrow). Day 3 was about making the air that enters your home as clean as possible; this chapter is about taking on the airborne allergens that circulate in your home. I'm talking about the dust that settles on and into your pillows, blankets, rugs, and other household furnishings. The molds and fungi that creep and crawl through the crevices of your apartment. The gunk and dirt that fills the nooks and seams of your basement.

But I'm not asking for a complete *home* makeover on top of your 7-Day Allergy Makeover. One makeover is enough for now. While you may need to get a few things, today will actually be more about getting rid of things you already own. Sometimes, having *too many* things can be bad for your allergies. Yes, that's right, it's time to cut down on the clutter!

The changes in this chapter are very budget friendly. But before we get to them, let's take a look at just what we can expect to find lurking in your living environment.

Dust

When it comes to allergies in the home, many people think dust is the problem. That's only half true—no, make that 2 percent true. You see, about 98 percent of what we call dust inside the home is simply skin that has flaked off *us*. It's that other 2 percent that poses a real problem. Dust contains, along with our skin and traces of fabric from the clothes we wear, other particles that are aller-genic. Pet dander and the droppings from insects and arachnids are the real culprits in your home. So let's spend the next few sections on them.

Dust Mites

Nature has made millions of beautiful animal species. But few people have any love for the dust mite. And with good reason. The thought of thousands of these microscopic arachnids swarming through every pillow and blanket they can find is probably enough to send a chill down even the most hardened allergy sufferer's spine. They live off flakes of dead human skin and reproduce within a brief two- to three-week lifespan. And the result of their short little lives? A lot of sneezing, wheezing, and harm to human health.

If you have dust mite allergies, you know exactly what a horror story living with them is. These little guys are marvelously adapted to live in our bedding and carpets, and some kinds of washings and cleanings aren't enough to get rid of them. Hint: To kill them, dry above 140°F. Their feces and even dead body parts contain enzymes that can cause IgE reactions (acute inflammatory responses) and can even lead to asthmatic symptoms. Itchy, watery eyes? Could be dust mites. Runny nose? Sneezing? Could be dust mites. Dust mite droppings (feces) are a part of that 2 percent of dust that isn't human skin, and they are part of the reason some people find themselves sneezing whenever dust gets kicked up.

Because dust mites prefer higher temperatures and high humidity, the midsummer months are the worst time of year, but they can plague you all year round. So if you're waking up and just not feeling right, it could be from a long night of breathing in what these creatures put out. Early morning runny nose and respiratory issues are often a good indication that you're sharing your bed with dust mites. Eliminating these mini spiders might be a huge key to your allergy health.

Cockroaches

If you think dust mites get little love, just ask anyone how they feel about cockroaches. These critters are so universally disliked, I almost feel bad for them—*almost*.

People with cockroach allergies can have severe asthmatic symptoms or rashes as well as the symptoms typical of IgE reactions. Fecal matter from cockroaches, much like that from dust mites, collects in the dust in your home and produces a whole host of allergic symptoms. Keeping food and trash well sealed and away from these roving scavengers is the best way to prevent an infestation. Look for any hidden water leakage. Cockroaches like damp, humid areas, such as under the sink or behind the dishwasher. If you have cockroaches, by all means, do your best to get rid of them naturally. Call your landlord or a "green" pest control company to get rid of the infestation. Clean your home well, especially your carpets and upholstery, where droppings from cockroaches and dust mites can settle.

Pet Dander

Contrary to popular belief, it's not animal *hair* that causes allergies; it's the dander—the dead skin that flakes off our pets—that causes runny nose, itchy eyes, coughing, and sneezing in allergy sufferers. Dander is what settles into dust around the home. Proteins in the skin or even in the animals' saliva can cause allergies for those who are sensitive. That's why kissing pets or letting them lick you is a definite no-no. (Also, microbes and parasites can be found in their saliva—not what you need.) Some types of cats and dogs are less allergenic, so if you're going to get a new one, it's worth looking into those breeds. You can find plenty of information online. But don't fret—you don't have to give away your beloved pup even if he is full of allergens. Keeping your pets clean and well groomed will go a long way toward helping your symptoms. If, on the other hand, you let the hair grow and don't clean your pet, the dander may agitate your symptoms while also feeding the dust mites that thrive on animal and human skin—perpetuating another vicious circle.

Mold

Mold is not part of the dust story, but it is one of the biggest sources of allergens in the home. Mold gets to you a little more indirectly than dust. Molds release spores, which travel through the air and eventually find their way into your respiratory system, much as pollen grains do after being released by flowering plants.

Yet molds vary. Some release their spores in the day; others at night, so there is no safe time that's free from mold. I'll give you tips for fending off the molds already in your home, but don't forget that plenty of mold comes from outside. Part of the reason for keeping your windows shut at night (and keeping those filters and ducts clean) is precisely to reduce the numbers of these airborne spores.

And it's true that some mold gives fair warning. That bluish-white fuzzy stuff on your bread is mold. So is that black slime in the crevices and grout between your shower tiles, and the white stuff that grows in your garden soil. And that mold could be what's causing your runny nose, itchy, watery eyes, fatigue, irritability, and other allergy symptoms.

If only all mold were so obvious. But mold can grow in your bath mat, rugs, humidifiers, closets, basement, or garage. It can grow on your bathroom ceiling as water vapor condenses up there. Mold can grow in your air ducts, too, as we talked about in the last chapter. But the key thing to remember is that mold grows *any-where* that gets wet and humid. That means it's especially impor-tant to take care of the humidity levels in your bathroom and keep things like towels and toothbrushes stored away so *they* don't col-lect mold, too.

Finally, though mold is everywhere, much of it is harmless to most people. Still, anyone with sensitivities should try to reduce their exposure to it as much as possible. That's why I put cheese, peanuts, and mushrooms on my list of foods to avoid. After all, if you're sensitive to mold, why eat it?

YOUR ACTION PLAN

If you have your air purifier in place, much of the dust and mold will be taken care of. If you still haven't bought yours yet, now is a good time to redouble your search. But an air purifier alone isn't enough for a whole-house allergy cleaning. What's more, an air purifier isn't going to suck the dust mites out of your bed and pil-lows. For that, we'll need to try a different approach. I'm also going to reiterate just how important it is to avoid plastics and anything with VOCs in it. These can lead to brain fog and fatigue. Elimi-nating plastics from your home (or, at minimum, storing them in the garage) is especially important if you have children. I'll explain exactly what to be on the lookout for.

Step 1: Upgrade Your Bed; Upgrade Your Sleep

Who doesn't love a good night's sleep? Sleep should mean relaxing dreams and a time for the body to recharge. When we wake up in the morning, we want to feel refreshed, recharged, and ready for day ahead—and without needing coffee!

Simply getting *enough* sleep is one of the best things you can do for your allergies. The deeper you sleep, the faster your body can recover and heal your allergy symptoms. The body needs time to process all the dust, dirt, chemicals, smoke, smog, pollen, mold, and *stress* it encounters during the day. Good sleep is what allows you to do that. Most people need between eight and nine hours of sleep. But with hectic work schedules, family duties, social obligations, and all the technological gadgetry we're plugged into, a restful night's sleep is more often a miracle than an everyday occurrence.

And if you have allergies on top of all that, restful sleep is something you may not have had in *years*. This is what I hear from countless patients. And my heart goes out to all of them. If you're not getting good sleep, dust mites are often to blame. If your bedding is filled with them, that's seven to nine hours each night you're breathing in allergens. Forgetting to clean sheets and pillows regularly means that more allergens will settle in your bedroom, ready to be inhaled. That's why upgrading your sleep begins with upgrading your bedding.

1. ELIMINATE DUST MITES. Pillows are dust mite apartment complexes. They're rent free and provide all the food these critters can eat—namely, your skin. Mattresses, too. They're the Ritz, where dust mites can live in luxury.

Simply put, your bedding provides an ideal environment for dust mites to burrow, eat, defecate, and make lots of baby mites. Some people can develop an itchy rash from dust mite allergies. But more likely are upper respiratory issues. If you're waking up congested, sneezing, or groggy, let's get rid of these bugs! Make the following action item a top priority.

Action item. Buy dust mite covers for your pillows, mattress, and duvet cover. You can buy these at any home-furnishing store.

Pillow covers usually run less than $20, and the mattress cover is only a bit more. Even though they're inexpensive, they are very effective. Be sure to wash them regularly with hot water. Dust mite covers have two main functions. First, they keep the dust mites in the pillow and make it impossible for them to get *to* your skin flakes. This essentially deprives them of their food source, starving them to death. Second, because it's not only the feces of live dust mites but the body parts of dead ones that are allergenic, the dust mite covers keep *everything* having to do with these bugs out of the air that you breathe. By trapping everything inside the cover, you won't inhale any of the proteins that these critters emit.

If you don't have a rubber allergy, latex pillows may be an option for you. Latex pillows are known to slow down the growth of dust mites and are considered dust mite resistant.

2. GET THE ALLERGENS OFF YOUR PILLOWS. When you lie down at night and put your head on the pillow, what else are you bringing with you? How about everything that touched your hair anytime during the day? Pollen, car exhaust, dust, chemicals. That's right, anything that gets in your hair or on your clothes can end up on your pillow. Being so close to your nose, the pillow provides a convenient platform for allergens to enter your respiratory system.

If you wear perfumes or if your shampoo contains chemicals, these collect on your pillows, and you'll be inhaling them all night long. That's why it's important to avoid toxic chemicals in your hygiene regimen. Along with reducing the amount of toxic chemicals you use on your body (see "Day 6: Clean Up Your Body"), *wash your pillowcases at least once a week* to remove airborne allergens.

And an important final note about pillows: I've had countless patients who have a particular emotional attachment to a favorite pillow. For some, that special pillow has been around for years and years—literally, since their teens! If this sounds like you, or even if you have a pillow that's more than two years old, now's the time to get a new one. After a couple of years (let alone a couple of decades!), the buildup of dust mites, bacteria, and mold is just too much. Time to let go and breathe easy.

Acid Reflux . . . Maybe

Tom came into my office with symptoms of acid reflux that came on only during the night, as an irritating cough that made sleeping difficult. He had suffered from this problem for more than ten years. His internist diagnosed it as acid reflux and prescribed an antacid (proton pump inhibitor). Tom took the drug faithfully for many years to stop the stomach acid production, but he just wasn't getting any relief from it. Finally, a year before seeing me, he stopped taking the drug because his respiratory symptoms were getting worse. The restless nights of coughing and poor sleep were now also affecting his wife's health and well-being. I took a detailed history of his eating habits and found that he was actually a very health-conscious person. He ate a diet free of gluten, sugar, and dairy, didn't eat late at night, didn't drink alcohol, and lived a retired, relatively stress-free existence. In short, his history did not reveal the usual reflux triggers.

My medical-detective side knew that his reflux symptoms just didn't match the diagnosis. He experienced the coughing fits only at night, so I asked him in detail about his sleeping hygiene and nightly ritual. He always slept on the same side of the bed, with his *favorite pillow*. Finally, I had zeroed in on the culprit to his coughing fits. He loved sleeping with this pillow that he had had for (no kidding) twenty-five years—ever since he got married. He mentioned that the pillow was all mis-shapen, "denser," and smelled "old," but he just couldn't bear to throw it away, because of its sentimental value. I asked him to consider getting a new one because the twenty-five-year-old pillow was probably infested with dust mites, bacteria, mold, viruses, and more. He was very resistant at first, but with some gentle coaxing from his wife, they both picked out new hypoallergenic pillows the next day. The results were nothing short of miraculous—within a week, Tom's coughing went away completely, and he was getting eight full hours of sleep. He also said he was snoring less, which made his wife very happy!

3. GET THE ALLERGENS OFF YOUR SHEETS. Think pillows collect a lot of allergens? How about your sheets? Everything that touches your skin during the day can get transferred to your sheets. Every chemical that is in the air (including sulfur dioxide or VOCs from furniture), all the microbes you touch (which can have a negative impact on your gut health), all the pollen that lands on your skin—all this stuff follows you home. If you drive on a smoggy day those chemicals can get trapped in your hair or on your skin if they aren't ingested directly. That can add up to a whole lot of chemicals and allergens! This is part of the reason why a shower before bedtime is such a good idea, as discussed on Day 6. By taking a shower *before* crawling into bed, you wash away the pollen, dust, sweat, chemicals, smoggy residue and even some of the bad bacteria that collect on your body. Don't forget to blow your nose as well. You will feel cleaner, more relaxed and less itchy—and ready for a more restful sleep. If you don't rinse your body off, those allergens may end up on your pillow, where you are very likely to inhale them causing middle-of-the night sneezing fits or nasal congestion. Before lying down, get those allergens and microbes off you so that you breathe in only the fresh HEPA-purified air. Even if you take a shower before bedtime, stick to the once-a-week (at minimum) laundering of all sheets, pillowcases, and bedding. Just in case something from outside makes it to your bedsheets, it won't linger for long.

Another good reason to launder sheets and bedding is because most of us sweat a bit during the night. While we rest, we rejuvenate our cells and organs and release metabolic waste, chemicals, and toxins through our sweat glands. So while it may seem like a hassle, the weekly cleaning is well worth it. Be sure to use mild, chemical-free detergents. When selecting new linens, the best materials are cotton, bamboo, hemp, and other natural, plant-based fabrics. Organic would be preferable.

4. TIME FOR A NEW MATTRESS? Dust mites don't live only on your pillows; they *love* mattresses. The older your mattress is, the more of these creatures have lived, spawned, and died in it. I recommend switching it out every five to seven years. Not only will you get rid of the dust mites, but a new mattress can also help you in your goal of getting better sleep.

If you already have a latex mattress, you may be able to go longer without switching it out because these are dust-mite resistant. For this reason, a latex mattress, just like a latex pillow, is a good choice if you're in the market for a new one. If you have a latex allergy, look for a mattress that is made of a hypoallergenic material, possibly 100 percent cotton or wool. When picking out a new mattress, avoid those treated with fire-retardant chemicals (meaning most commercial mattresses) because these can produce all types of allergy symptoms. In some cases, to get an untreated mattress, you may have to ask for a doctor's note and give it to the manufacturer.

Action item. Wash your sheets and pillows at least once a week. Replace your pillows if you have had them for more than two years. Replace your mattress if you have had it more than five to seven years.

Step 2: Allergy-Proof Your Bedroom

Now that we've taken care of your bed, it's time to make the rest of your bedroom a safe haven from allergies. If you're like most people, your bedroom probably has some of your most cherished items: photos and knickknacks, presents from loved ones, memorabilia from high school or college.

Your picture of Grandma probably isn't kicking up your allergies. But what about all those books and magazines collecting dust? Or those heaps of clothes in the closet that don't even fit anymore? At the end of the day, there are several things you may want to take out of your bedroom if you're serious about allergy-proofing your home. It's another case of less is more.

1. PETS. When deciding what to keep out of the bedroom, we'll start with the hardest things first: our pets. Some of us are so attached to our pets, we can't *imagine* sleeping without them on the bed, on top of the pillow, or even on top of *us*.

Remember, your pet's dander and saliva can be intense allergy catalysts. When you're inhaling your puppy's dander and skin flakes all through the night, your nose and throat will not be at their best. Congestion, runny nose, and itchy eyes will become an unwelcome part of your morning reality. Make your bedroom, and those precious eight hours of sleep, sacred. Put your pets in another room for the night.

2. PLANTS. Remember our discussion of mold a few pages back? Many of those spores can come from natural mold growth in the soil of your potted plants. Instead of keeping your plants in the house, why not give them to a trusted friend who *doesn't* suffer from allergies? The plants will brighten your friend's day without the sneezing and itchy eyes, nasal congestion, and irritation.

3. BOOKS AND MAGAZINES. Book lovers, take heed! Your beloved collection might be at the root of your allergy symptoms. Not only does dust settle on them, but books are prone to collecting mold. Even the inks in books—and especially in glossy magazines—can cause allergies. Magazines are also notorious for their perfumed interiors filled with synthetic chemicals. Headaches, grogginess, runny nose, wheezing, and sore throat are only some of the symptoms I've seen in my patients.

Don't become the victim of your love of knowledge. Keep the books if you like, but keep them out of the bedroom. Even better, sell them to a local bookstore, donate what you can, or give them away to nonallergic friends. Reducing clutter is not just good for allergies—it's emotionally and psychologically liberating!

4. WINDOW TREATMENTS AND COVERINGS. Dust, dust, and more dust. It can seem to be everywhere. Another little spot for dust to collect is on your curtains, shades, and blinds. Dust and clean them regularly.

On a related note, to improve your sleep, I recommend getting blackout curtains or shades, which will eliminate up to 99 percent of ambient light. The darker your room, the better sleep you will get. When your body falls into a deeper sleep, this will make it easier to calm your nervous system and relax the "sympathetic dominant" state in which we spend so much of our lives. And when you wake up, you'll be less sensitive to allergens because your body has had time to repair and heal itself.

You'd be surprised by how much more restful it is to sleep in true darkness (with clean, well-maintained curtains, of course)!

5. SKELETONS OUT OF THE CLOSET! Nearly all of us have some closet clutter we can get rid of. It will help you eliminate dust from your closet, and give you a renewed commitment to the clothes you really love and want to wear. Even more important, dehumidify and ventilate your closets to prevent mold growth. Remember, mold can grow in any damp, humid environment. A dehumidifier will do the job; as an alternative, try calcium chloride pellets, which extract excess water from the air.

6. ELECTROMAGNETIC EXPOSURE. Another source of night-time irritation comes from our much-cherished devices: laptops, tablets, cell phones, video games, mp3 players—the list goes on and on. These devices emit electromagnetic radiation that can—especially when placed near your body—disrupt your natural sleep cycles and immune system. If you're not sleeping deeply, check to see that all these devices are turned *off* at night. If you need an alarm clock, just turn your phone to airplane mode and use its built-in alarm.

I also recommend putting everything that uses electricity in your room—including lamps, stereos, and computers—on a single surge protector so that you can flip them *all* off with a single button. Power down your gadgets, and your body will find it easier to power down, too. When you crawl into bed, avoid the electric blanket! At night, zero electricity is really the way to go. Before you know it, you won't want to sleep any other way.

Action item. Remove all animals, plants, books, and magazines out of your bedroom. Donate plants and extra books. Dehumidify your closets. Get complete blackout shades and keep them dust-free. Turn off all electronic devices and appliances in the bedroom.

Teenage Insomnia

Tiffany came to my office after going to several doctors to find out why she had been suffering from chronic insomnia for the past two years. It took her over an hour to fall asleep each night, and once asleep, she would wake up every couple of hours. After tossing and turning throughout the night, she would wake up feeling as though she hadn't slept a wink. With a heavy workload as a high school junior and the star player on the basketball team, Tiffany worried that it all was catching up to her. What with being constantly tired and irritable and catching colds every other month, she actually thought she had mononucleosis, a viral infection that young people in high school often get. After doing a blood test that ruled out mononucleosis, I studied her daily sleep hygiene. She took her shower after basketball practice, ate dinner, finished her homework, and was in bed by 9:45 or 10:00 p.m. Unremarkable so far. I asked if she had to use an alarm clock to wake up, and that was when the most important clue turned up. She mentioned that she used her cell phone alarm to wake her up at 6:45 a.m. When I asked her where she put her phone—whether she kept it on the nightstand or her desk—she confessed that she always put it under her pillow, under her head. And it was on all night just in case one of her best friends should text her. She had gotten her cell phone her freshman year, and this was her nightly ritual; hence the two years of no sleep! I tried not to react too dramatically, but her mother was just as surprised as I was. I educated Tiffany about electromagnetic and microwave radiation emitted from cell phones and how it can disrupt the brain, physical growth, and sleep patterns. Then I gave her immediate instructions to put the cell phone on airplane mode whenever she turned on her alarm. Most important, she had to get it out of her bed and put it on her desk, which was seven feet away. Two weeks later, she came dancing into my office, full of energy, and gave me a big hug. She was getting eight hours of uninterrupted deep sleep, and she was starting to love life again.

Step 3: What's in Your Child's Bedroom?

If you're concerned about your child's allergy health, start by making the right choices in the bedroom. Just as in your own bedroom, move all plants and books out of there, keep the closets ventilated, and make sure the curtains and bedding stay especially clean. In addition to these changes, there are a few extra things you'll want to pay special attention to.

To make the bedroom a safe and comfortable place for your children, follow these steps.

1. PLASTIC TOYS. Most of us grew up with plastic dolls or action figures. But the truth is out, and the evidence for plastic toys is not looking good. Plastics (and this includes your plastic kitchenware, by the way) leach xenoestrogenic chemicals, which are known endocrine disruptors—altering the normal functioning of hormones in the body. Breathing in the fumes emanated by plastics is bad enough. But children—as I'm sure you've learned by now if you have any—love to chew on anything they can.

Teething on plastic toys, especially those with bisphenol A (BPA), greatly increases the rate of exposure to these harmful endocrine disruptors. Constant exposure to plastics is not good for respiratory and hormonal health. It can also cause brain fog and poor concentration. There are, however, wonderful BPA-free toys that are just as fun and allergy free. Anything that is all natural, such as cotton or most woods, is better than plastic. Work toward eliminating plastic toys altogether. And beware of the packaging itself. Because most toys come wrapped in plastic, be sure to air them out before giving them to your kids, to give the toxic fumes time to outgas.

2. STUFFED TOYS. Everyone loves a good teddy bear, right? While I would never say to eliminate these toys altogether, it is smart to reduce the number of stuffed toys in your home. Like pillows, stuffed animals attract dust and dust mites and can contribute to sneezing and runny noses. If you do have a lot of stuffed toys, pick a special place for them, away from where your children spend most of their time. Above all, be sure to keep the stuffed animals out of the bedroom. Otherwise, the cost may well be hours spent inhaling dust mite proteins. Let your children play with these toys in the living room, a playroom, or another area far from where they sleep. Also, wash and pop them in the dryer regularly to reduce dust, mold, and mite content.

Action item. For teething babies, use BPA-free chewing toys. For older children, replace plastic toys with nontoxic wooden ones; minimize stuffed animals and keep them out of the bedroom.

Step 4: Make the Living Room Livable

Sofas, carpets, rugs, floors—these are natural havens for dust, mold, and mites. Besides regular cleanings, let's see what else you can do to allergy-proof your living room.

1. FURNITURE. Shelves and furniture are among the few cases where older may actually be better for your home. Older furniture has spent years outgassing. That is, the chemicals in the glues and finishes have evaporated and are not as harmful to your health. Newer furniture will often contain the VOCs we talked about in in the last chapter. And those VOCs can mean headaches, sluggishness, foggy brain, and a whole host of other allergy symptoms.

If you have furniture made of particleboard and laminated wood, be especially careful. Formaldehyde and toluene are prevalent in these materials. Anything with glues and adhesives will have volatile organic compounds and other chemicals.

When choosing furniture, stick with the stuff made of real wood, glass, natural stone, clay, and iron. Use your allergy makeover as a convenient excuse to go to the thrift store or antiques store and take a gander. I found much of my favorite living room and office furniture at the well-known Santa Monica flea market: antique cabinets, travertine coffee tables, Asian art, and more.

2. FLOOR COVERINGS. Nothing ties a room together like a nice rug. But then again, nothing traps dust like an old rug or carpet! Vacuum and clean all you want—there's still a high likelihood of dust mites burrowing in them.

If you have carpet, I strongly recommend that you check out what's underneath. Often, you'll have a nice wood floor that's just waiting to help you toward an allergy-free lifestyle. Natural wood won't irritate your nasal passages nearly as much as dust mites. Tear up that carpet and liberate the floor beneath!

But keep in mind that not all woods are created equal. Some people are very sensitive to certain types of wood. Terpenes—a set of compounds found in tree resins—can affect many allergy sufferers. These are especially prevalent in coniferous trees, so it's best to avoid them when putting in a new floor. Also, the phenols in many trees can cause problems. Phenols are a naturally occurring toxin that can be found in poison ivy and poison oak as well as more innocuous plants. However, many types of wood also have naturally occurring phenols that, when inhaled, can be disruptive to your body. Lethargy and fatigue are common symptoms, and the low-energy states they produce can be quite pronounced if you have a high sensitivity.

If you want the best odds of avoiding allergic flare-ups, I

recommend using natural stone or tile flooring. Natural stone and tile floorings include travertine, slate, terra-cotta, and marble. Ask your contractor to use a thin-set mortar (the cement material that bonds the tile to the floor) that is VOC free.

If you are renting, the situation is a bit different because you probably won't have the luxury of tearing up your carpet or installing a stone floor. If you have carpet, vacuum regularly with a HEPA vacuum cleaner. Like the air purifier, it will pick up particles down to microscopic levels, and while it can't eliminate everything, it will go a long way toward making your carpet more allergy friendly. In fact, everyone can benefit from using a HEPA-filter vacuum. You can even use it on furniture and wood floors to remove invisible particles that might be agitating your nose, throat, and eyes. When you clean rugs and carpets, the best method is simply to steam them or use hot water. If you do use cleaning agents, be careful to use only mild, all-natural cleaners to avoid your risk of exposure to toxic chemicals.

3. GOING SHOELESS. Another way to keep allergens out of your home entirely is to avoid tracking them in, in the first place. Many Asian households, including that of my Korean family, have long used this sensible practice. When you walk around during the day, your shoes pick up dirt, bacteria, pollen, and countless other things (including some we'd rather not name). If you wear your shoes around the house, you're simply spreading these over your floor. Eventually, they'll find their way into your lungs or even your digestive system. The no-shoes policy is especially important if you have infants and toddlers. Because young children spend so much time on the floor, touching and licking everything in reach, there's a high probability that your child will find an allergen or two during the day.

4. WHAT TO LOOK FOR IN A NEW HOME. This tip applies only to prospective renters and home buyers. If you know you're allergy prone, don't you want a home that's been as well maintained and allergen free as possible? Carpeted apartments that were home to smokers with dogs and cats, replete with moldy bathrooms, are best avoided.

Ask about the previous inhabitants. Did they have pets? Did they smoke? Any previous water damage? A leaky pipe or a flooded toilet? Don't just ask—poke around, too. Check the bathrooms, especially the ceilings, to see if there's mold. If you see cracking, or the walls are buckling or puckering, it's often a sign of water damage. That means a higher chance of mold and mold spores. A bathroom window or a fan is essential so that you can dehumidify it and air it out.

And perhaps most important, listen to your gut. Do you *feel* comfortable in your prospective new abode? Can you breathe without straining? Do your eyes feel moist and comfortable instead of itchy and watery? Do you sneeze a lot? And what about the emotional vibe? Does it feel like a place of rest and revitalization? Your intuition will give you a good sense of just how comfortable your body feels in a new place. Make sure your new home really feels like a place where you can see yourself living allergy free.

Action item. Look for nontoxic wood and iron furniture as well as antiques that have already outgassed. Natural stone, tile, and terra-cotta flooring are best for allergies. Wooden floors are first runner up. Leave shoes at the door. When looking for a new apartment, be an allergy detective and ask questions.

Step 5: Garden Nature's Way

Your backyard is a great place to surround yourself with your favorite plants and herbs. You may be able to move indoor plants outside, if they are capable of surviving. And if you decide you want to grow your own vegetables and fruits, all the better (organic and *very* locally grown!).

That said, be careful not to use toxic pesticides or chemical agents on any of your plants, including your landscaping and lawn. These toxins can drift into your home. Diatomaceous earth is often enough to take care of ants, fleas, spiders, and slugs. This powder made of fossilized diatoms (hard-shelled algae) kills the insects by a mechanical means of pest control rather than a toxic chemical one. Diatomaceous earth cuts into the slug or the insect exoskeleton and dehydrates it. Do find one that is considered food grade, so you can use it indoors as well as outdoors. And do wear a mask while you sprinkle the powder in corners, crevices, and other dark places where insects roam—you don't want to inhale it accidentally and cause more allergy symptoms!

Many types of plants actually repel insects. For example, if you do companion planting of basil with tomatoes, the basil will help the growth and flavor of the tomatoes, as well as repel mosquitoes and flies. You can go on the Web and learn more about the principles of permaculture and other forms of pest control used in organic gardening. There's quite a bit of literature on the subject, and it's fun to design your garden with plant synergies in mind.

Be careful with fertilizers. Dogs and other animals that romp in the yard can absorb the chemicals through their feet, and these can be potentially harmful to skin, mucous membranes, and kidneys. Children playing in the backyard are also vulnerable to the chemicals in the garden, so know what you're putting there.

Action item. Do not use pesticides, herbicides, or fungicides. Minimize use of fertilizer.

DAY 5

CLEAN UP YOUR
KITCHEN

Besides the living room, the kitchen is often the most popular room in the house. And if there's a really good cook around, it's likely *the* most popular spot of all.

In recent years, open kitchen design has become increasingly trendy, and it's not at all uncommon to have an hour-long conversation over a simmering pot of chicken soup or a tray of roasted beets. My point? The kitchen is not just a place where food gets cooked. Modern kitchens are, above all else, social spaces. And while the open kitchen has much to recommend it, it also means more exposure to a whole host of kitchen allergens that you might not suspect.

If there is one place in the house where molds, bacteria, and viruses can live it up, this is it. That's because there are so many things for them to feast on. With just a little neglect, your kitchen can become a petri dish for all sorts of microorganisms, and when these work their way into your food, it can be irritating. Your gut bioflora can be thrown off, microbes can produce respiratory issues, and you may even get sick. Not only are you exposed to them as airborne allergens but you are actually swallowing them whole. Proper food storage, cleaning, and disposal will be the guiding principles of allergy health in the kitchen. But even that isn't going to fix all the problems.

Proper kitchenware is a huge issue. Much of the kitchenware we use is better suited for recycling than for tossing a Mediterranean salad or sautéing broccolini. More and more of my patients are concerned with the health risks of nonstick cookware and plastic storage ware. But few understand why they should stop eating with metal utensils or start washing vegetables with vitamin C crystals. So not only will I give you some tips on how to fight bacteria and mold in the kitchen but I'll also help you get safer, nonchemically treated pots, pans, and utensils.

Finally, when it comes time to take on the month-old head of broccoli that's been transformed into a greenish-brown glop with several colors of furry growth, you may be tempted to reach for the bleach and chemical cleaners. But in the long run, this will only increase your exposure to chemical toxins, which can irritate your eyes, lungs, and digestive system. Nowhere is the balance between keeping the space clean and potentially *worsening* your toxic load so tenuous as in the kitchen. Coupled with the improved food choices you learned on Day 1, the kitchen makeover outlined in this chapter will ensure that your food is not only healthful, organic, and locally grown but also free of the molds and bacteria that can cause upset stomachs and allergic reactions.

THE ALLERGENS IN YOUR KITCHEN

First, let's take a look at some of the allergens you may be exposing yourself to in the kitchen.

Polytetrafluoroethylene (PTFE) and Nonstick Pans

If you have pans made with a nonstick coating called Teflon or polytetrafluoroethylene (PTFE), it's time to think deeply about whether that convenience is worth it. After reading this section, you may agree that it's time to find a better solution.

When scratched and heated, nonstick pans can release a chemical called perfluorooctanoic acid (PFOA). Most of the time, the scratches are caused by metal utensils. The best alternatives to metal forks and spatulas are wooden utensils, which won't scratch as much. Better yet, try not to use PTFE-coated nonstick pans at all!

PFOA is slow to leave the human body—that is, our tissues have a difficult time detoxing the chemical out; thus it builds up over time and adds to our overall toxic load. PFOA has been shown to cause liver damage and developmental problems in animals and is a known carcinogen. Public Health England agrees: "A range of toxic effects has been seen in animals following chronic exposure [to PFOA] including effects on the liver, gastrointestinal tract and thyroid hormone levels."[1]

If PFOA causes these problems in animals, there is a high likelihood that it will have similar adverse effects on humans as well. In fact, Public Health England goes so far as to assert, "A small number of occupational studies have reported an association between exposure to PFOA and PFOS [perfluorooctanesulfonic acid, a chemical similar to it] and several forms of cancer."[2] This means that workers involved in the production of PFOA have statistically significantly high rates of health issues, including cancer, than the general population.

But PFOA is more prevalent than you might think. It is also found in things like dental floss, carpet cleaners, and microwave popcorn bags, so be aware of it (and avoid it) in all its commercial uses. And there is one final place where you might find PFOA, which may surprise you: In your tap water! But PFOA is *not* yet regulated by the Safe Drinking Water Act (although it is under review as a candidate for regulation). Remember, no chemical has been added to that list in twenty years. Now, how glad are you that you bought that water purifier?

Plastics (Including BPA, Polystyrene, and PET)

The world uses plastics for countless things: toys, bottles, containers, cups, utensils. It's what our televisions and gaming consoles are made of; it's part of what helps our blenders blend and our lights switches switch. Nylon stockings? Plastic. Ties to keep the hair out of your eyes? Plastic. The latter half of the twentieth century may well be remembered as one great experiment with plastics.

I would like to think that perhaps the twenty-first century will be remembered as the century when we reduced the use of plastics as much as we could.

The first reason is environmental. Plastics are made mostly of petroleum and other fossil fuels. So while we may drive that eco-friendly car and buy organic vegetables, until we greatly reduce our dependence on plastics, we are not doing all we can to ease the environmental crisis. Fossil fuels are a precious resource, and we should find alternative resources.

And plastic does not break down for a very, very long time. This means that every water bottle we use, every wrapper we unwrap, piles up somewhere on this earth. Remember, *reuse* and *recycle* are only two parts of the green equation. When it comes to plastics, we should focus on *reduce*. Considering that twelve million tons of plastics are produced every year, you can see that we have a long way to go.

The second reason to avoid plastic is directly related to your allergy symptoms and overall health. Many of the plastics we use every day, including in the kitchen, are potentially carcinogenic and are known endocrine disruptors. I have seen my patients suffer from inexplicable brain fog, lethargy, and headaches. Others have itching skin, hives, and rashes. They suspect pollen, food allergens, and pets. And behind it all? Too much exposure to plastic. Plastic spatulas, plastic plates, plastic storage ware. When those patients rid themselves of plastic, they whisked away the allergies, too.

So let's look at some of the specific plastic compounds and the problems they may be causing you. There are different kinds of plastics, and they are identified by a number ranging from 1 to 7, in the center of a triangular "chasing arrow" symbol, usually found at the bottom of all plastic products. Knowing the differences will help you make better decisions on which plastics to choose and to recycle.

BISPHENOL A (PLASTIC 7). BPA is a chemical found in many plastics known as polycarbonates, including the plastic storage ware in your home. BPA is an endocrine disruptor that mimics estrogen (xenoestrogenic) and can lead to developmental issues in both genders. BPA exposure is especially risky during fetal development and infancy because the effects of hormones play a key role in body development.

University of Florida researcher Stephen Musson, however, claims that the risks of BPA exposure are important to consider at all times: "Laboratory studies conducted since the 1990s have noted that low-dose BPA exposure may be connected to abnormal penis development in males, early sexual maturation in females, an increase in neurobehavioral problems such as attention deficit hyperactivity disorder (ADHD) and autism, an increase in childhood and adult obesity and type 2 diabetes, and an increase in hormonally mediated cancers, such as prostate and breast cancers."[3]

For these reasons, BPA has been declared toxic by the Canadian department of the environment, although the government still allows it in kitchenware and household products. In the United States, the Food and Drug Administration (FDA) has banned its use in baby bottles because of the developmental risks it poses. Studies of rats have consistently verified these findings as well as BPA's carcinogenic effects. BPA's endocrine-disrupting qualities can contribute to your toxic load and make it more difficult for your body to handle other allergens.

So how does BPA get into your bloodstream? The kitchen! BPA can easily leach into food stored in plastic containers, especially if they are microwaved. Type 7 plastics are especially rife with BPA.

BPA is also in the lining of canned foods including soda, beer, vegetables, and soups. A few canned-food manufacturing companies voluntarily use BPA-free can linings. One particular company has been using BPA-free cans since 1999. We can hope more companies will soon change and label their cans "BPA free."

Plastic containers labeled 1, 2, and 5 are BPA free. Later in this chapter, we will go over the best alternatives for storing and cooking food so you can avoid exposure to BPA.

POLYSTYRENE FOAM (PLASTIC 6). Plastic foam products such as cups and clamshell takeout containers have a little number 6 inside the recycling triangle symbol. Polystyrene is easy to identify, and if you see that number, avoid it as much as possible. (Or, to make your life even easier, avoid plastics altogether.)

You may be asking, what's so bad about plastic foam? When you use it for foodstuff, toxic chemicals such as styrene leach out of the container and find their way into your diet. Hot foods and drinks are especially bad, as well as anything acidic, because heat and acid break down plastic. That means you are eating plastic. This effect is magnified if you microwave polystyrene foam—*something you should never do.* From an allergy perspective, plastic foam has been known to cause brain fog and confusion, but it can also agitate the eyes and skin. It can even cause depression, neurological issues, headaches, and gastrointestinal symptoms. Beyond all that, most of it is not recyclable, so it just adds to the pollution of the environment.

For some optimism about the fight against plastic foam, we need look no further than the work of a host of eleven-to-thirteen-year-olds in my own area. Los Angeles County, acceding to the demands of concerned middle school students, banned foam containers in its schools, which now use compostable lunch trays. In fact, California even considered a statewide ban of polystyrene foam, although it was shot down in the legislature. If our middle school students can ban these products, so can you! So next time you get a doggie bag, ask for paper or cardboard. And don't forget, even some eggs come in foam packaging. For your allergy health, be vigilant about plastic foam.

PET (PLASTIC 1). Many soda and water bottles, including the "reusable" water bottles popular with outdoor enthusiasts, are made of plastic 1, or polyethylene terephthalate (PET). Repeated use of PET bottles increases the risk of leaching toxins and bacterial growth. The former can slow our ability to process allergens, while the latter can destroy good bacteria, making it more difficult to cope with foods high in fermentable sugars.

And don't forget those ketchup and mustard bottles! Leonard Sax argues that despite previous beliefs to the contrary, PET plastics may pose hormonal risks: "Beverages and condiments in PET containers may be contaminated by endocrine-disrupting chemicals."[4]

Coffee Toxic?

Sara lived by the beach in Monterey, California, and had a new job in the housekeeping department at a beautiful local resort. She would arrive a half hour early just so she could relax with her second cup of coffee: the famous house brand that the hotel was known for. After a few weeks at her job, she started to feel tired and anxious at the same time, soon after she started her workday. She had trouble concentrating on her work. She thought it was that second shot of caffeine, so she switched to decaffeinated coffee, but it didn't make a difference. After a few more weeks, in addition to her fatigue and anxiety, she noticed numbness around her mouth, tongue, and throat.

Sarah got worried about her strange symptoms, so she went to her internist. The doctor wasn't sure, so she sent Sarah out for an MRI and a slew of blood tests. "Good news!" the doc said. "Nothing is wrong with you. All tests are normal." (My patients often get such statements from their doctors.) "Great, no pathology," Sarah said. "But how about my symptoms!"

Sarah drove six hours down the coast to my office to get some answers. After going over her history, I was puzzled by her symptoms. About 90 percent of the time, after hearing the patient's history, I already have a working diagnosis, but Sarah's case was not calling out to me. I asked all the right questions and performed a detailed physical exam—all unremarkable. I went over her history one more time, but this time I asked for her entire daily regimen: what time she woke up, what type of toothpaste she used, every detail of her breakfast, the type of coffee she drank at home, whether the stove was gas or electric, when and how she used the microwave, whether she pumped her own gas for the car, parked underground, touched any chemicals at the hotel. And then I asked, "What type of cup do you use at the hotel for that second cup of coffee?" She replied, "A medium-size white foam cup, filled with piping-hot decaf coffee." There it was! Polystyrene foam, which leaches the toxic chemical styrene, especially when used for hot drinks or soup.

I asked her to stop using the plastic foam cups and start using a regular ceramic or glass coffee mug. Then I put her on my 7-Day Allergy Makeover program to get the chemicals out of her body, reduce her anxiety, and regain her energy. This also included the oil-pulling technique (Day 6) to get the chemicals out of her mouth (including her tongue and throat) and get rid of the numbness. I asked her to come back in two weeks, after she completed her detox regimen.

After five days on my allergy makeover, Sarah called me to say that her anxiety was dissipating, she was starting to feel more energy, and although her mouth still felt odd, she hoped the numbness would be gone soon. Two weeks later, the mouth and tongue numbness were gone and she felt more vibrant and full of energy. And to top it off, she was seven pounds lighter!

Sarah asked her manager at the hotel to consider changing the cups for the employees to paper cups, and after hearing about her medical case, the manager made it happen. Soon after the hotel switched to paper cups, Monterey County banned the use of all takeout polystyrene containers and cups by local restaurants and other establishments. A healthful decision.

Notice the last two syllables of PET's full chemical name: *phthalate*. I want to caution you about this toxin. Phthalates, often called *plasticizers* due to their stretchability, are hormone-disrupting chemicals commonly found in plastic but also in a wide range of everyday personal care products, which we'll learn about in the next chapter. These include synthetic perfumes, eye shadow, moisturizers, body washes, nail polish, and hair spray; the enteric coatings of pharmaceutical tablets; children's toys; and even fatty foods such as butter, milk, and meat products.[5]

Indeed, they are so ubiquitous that most Americans have several different phthalates in their urine.[6] Studies have shown that American men with abdominal obesity or diabetes were more likely to have high levels of the phthalate metabolites in their urine than men without those problems.[7] Obesity and diabetes are two very common chronic illnesses today, and if avoiding phthalates might be a way to prevent or reverse them, what are we waiting for?

YOUR KITCHEN MAKEOVER

While very few people truly enjoy cleaning the kitchen (if you are one of them, you are lucky), we have tried to simplify the process here and focus on the most important things you can do for your allergies. A good deal of my instructions will also involve eliminating those hidden allergens you never knew contributed to your allergy symptoms.

Step 1: Clean Your Refrigerator

How often do you clean your refrigerator? I once did a survey with over a hundred of my patients, and the average frequency for cleaning their fridge was every two months. If you could only see with the naked eye all the bacteria, yeasts, molds, and slime molds in your fridge, you would definitely schedule your fridge cleanups every week.

Let's be honest: doing laundry, washing dishes, scrubbing your floors, and even scraping mold out of the shower grout are probably more fun than cleaning the fridge. You have to pull out every container, throw away that three-week old broccoli-shaped science experiment in the crisper, inspect four half-empty bottles of ketchup, and come face-to-face with slimy shelves and drawers. Then you have to take everything out and wash it by hand if it doesn't fit in the dishwasher. Meanwhile, everyone has to go rummaging through grocery bags full of disorganized foodstuffs, asking you where you put that half-eaten orange from lunch yesterday. You're wiping down every nook, cranny, crevice, and corner of the fridge, all the while knowing that it's bound to be back to this state mere days from now. It's frustrating.

But remember, this is your health we're talking about. Bacteria and mold spreading to the food you eat is simply too big a risk to your gut health and digestive allergies for you not to be concerned with the cleanliness of this space. That's why, if you want your food to be as fresh and uncontaminated as possible, you simply must clean your fridge *at least once a week*.

I know it can be a daunting task, but I have some good news. By cleaning the fridge the all-natural way, you will reduce the amount of time you spend with food all over the counters, and a grimy sponge in your hand. In fact, you might not even need to do a complete overhaul while you clean. Let's look at exactly what you need to do to take care of your fridge.

First, throw away all suspect vegetables. That rubbery kale? Chuck it. That slightly browning bag of salad mix? Out. It's especially important to toss greens and herbs that have been stored in your fridge for more than three or four days. I generally will not eat anything that has been in fridge for more than three days. Mold spores and bacteria love feeding on older fruits and vegetables. That is what they do in nature: they are the decomposers.

They break down vegetation. It's a natural part of the wonderful ecosystem, and nothing goes to waste. You just don't want the harmful microorganisms in your fresh food; otherwise, you or your family will be subject to a possible stomachache, gas and bloating, or untimely trips to the bathroom!

Not only that, but as we learned on Day 1, having the right balance of healthful bioflora in the gut is essential for digesting good FODMAP foods like beans, cabbage, and broccoli. Harmful bacteria in the gut kill off the beneficial ones. Cleaning your fruits and vegetables is not just good for removing the bad—it's essential for preserving the good.

One more thing: Before tossing out the spoiled veggies or fruit, don't open the bag for one last daring whiff to see if they might still be edible. That ill-considered inhalation will get your nose full of the very mold spores and gases you are trying to avoid. Better to just toss it.

If we were to summarize this rule, it's very simple: *Always eat and cook fresh veggies.*

Think about it. Our ancestors walked eight to ten miles a day picking berries from the brambles and picking edible nuts and fruits from the tree. Everything they ate came right off the vine, bush, or branch, or straight from Mother Earth. Their diet was varied, local, and almost never "preserved" in any way. While hunting and gathering probably wouldn't suit many of us as a lifestyle choice, there is an important lesson to learn: fresh, local, and organic is what our bodies were made for.

A lot of my patients feel very wasteful when first following this advice. If you find yourself throwing away lots of vegetables, here's what I suggest: next time you go grocery shopping, buy less produce at one time; then go to the store more often. Instead of that massive once-a-week shopping trip, why not do two or three quick trips during the week? Why not find a weekend farmers' market so you can not only get ripe, recently picked veggies and fruits, all grown nearby, but also enjoy the sunshine and being outdoors while you shop?

Second, instead of trashing the expired veggies, put them to a better use in your own backyard composter. Some compost makers are small and discrete for the balcony of a small apartment dwelling. Use it to make natural fertilizer for your garden and plants. It's all a win–win.

Fruits are a slightly different story. Many fruits can last longer than vegetables—some for two weeks or even longer. In nature, their role is to help spread the seeds by remaining attractive to animals and insects as long as possible. Leave an apple and a bowl of spinach on the counter and tell me which one looks edible after a week. Still, if you have any doubts, err on the side of caution and toss your fruit into the composter.

Next time you go grocery shopping, buy less produce at one time.

But above all, do not become an unwitting mold eater. You want to get nutrients and vitamins, not mold spores and slime, out of your fruits and vegetables. As we mentioned on Day 1, berries and grapes often have mold in the box or bag even before you bring them home. If you put them in one of the fruit storage bins of your fridge, you're bound to contaminate the rest of the fruits or vegetables in the same storage bin. Bring home fruits with a tough skin, such apples, pears, watermelon, and citrus fruits, and wash them with vitamin C crystals before refrigerating them (as explained later in the chapter).

This process will help keep your produce fresh and crisp and will remove many of the mold and bacteria that settle on them.

Before we get there, we're going to go look at everything that has been packaged. This doesn't mean you can never buy packaged items; it simply means that most fridges have too much packaged clutter: hummus containers and mustard jars (often plastic), long-forgotten salad dressing and cocktail sauce, and now impossible-to-find varieties of blueberry jam.

If any of these are expired or even close to the expiration date, get them out of the fridge! The best plan is to empty and rinse out the bottles and jars and put them with the recycling. Many of us love to buy the double-super-duper-size bottles of ketchup or mayo that are made with sugar and preservatives. Sure, it saves a few cents, but in the long run, it costs you more by harming your health. Unless you are into hot dog-eating competitions, you probably won't be using enough of these condiments quickly enough to avoid turning them into brewery vats for mold and bacteria. If you want to keep buying these types of condiments, always buy smaller bottles or jars. And remember to buy glass, not plastic. Better yet, use that trip to the farmers' market to get some fresh herbs and spices and mix up a salad dressing of your own. Not only is it fresher than anything you'll find in a store but I bet it will taste better than most of those mass-produced varieties! Keep it simple and organic with fresh basil, herbs, olive oil, sea salt, pepper, and white balsamic vinegar, and you'll never go wrong. I've done it for years, and I can eat it any day of the week. Same thing with mayonnaise and ketchup. If our grandparents made them from scratch, so can we, without the chemicals and preservatives.

Now that you've eliminated those less-than-garden-fresh veggies and those not-so-recently-bought jars of condiments, your weekly fridge cleaning is going to become a lot easier. But the very last thing you want to do to your fridge—*the place where you store the food you eat*—is pump it full of bleach and chemicals with unpronounceable names. Put those toxins in an enclosed environment with your food, and you're doing more harm than good.

That's why this last tip is not only better for your allergies but time saving as well. When fridge-cleaning time rolls around next (right after you read this chapter—*wink, wink*), use a simple solution of white distilled vinegar and water (half vinegar and half water in a spray bottle). Wear dishwashing gloves, and with a clean towel or sponge, wipe down all your shelves and drawers with this mix. The bacteria and mold will recoil in horror . . . and die. Remember, there was a time, in your grandmothers' or great-grandmothers' time, when all the fancy soaps and sprays didn't exist. What did our families use? There's a good chance it was this very mixture—it's a time-tested formula that works.

Best of all, because vinegar is just another natural food product, you don't necessarily have to remove everything from the fridge each time you clean it. You can simply take a paper towel or sponge and wipe down everything without launching a full-on archaeological excavation of your foodstuffs. Of course, at least once a month, you still should take everything out and wipe down your fridge. When you do this thorough monthly cleaning, use hot water and ecofriendly soap for the drawers and shelves, and air-dry them completely before putting them back in. By doing more regular cleanings with the water-and-vinegar mix, you will save yourself a lot of hassle in the long run. You'll save time, avoid chemicals, and get less exposure to mold and bacteria.

Action item. Throw away all old produce and recycle expired condiment jars and bottles. Clean your refrigerator once a week with the vinegar-and-water solution.

Step 2: Clean Your Food Properly

So you're buying organic food, taking it home, and running it under that stream of reverse osmosis filtered water from your faucet before you eat it. Everything's good, right? I wish I could say yes.

While what you're doing is already miles ahead of how most Americans treat their food, we want to put you in the upper echelon of allergy-free households. The truth is, very few of us know how to clean and store our fruits, vegetables, grains, nuts, and dried beans properly.

So let's start with the facts. Organic food reduces the risk of pesticides, herbicides, and fungicides, which is great. However, even organic foods can be exposed to these contaminants via "drift" from other farms. Because locally grown food spends little time in trucks or on shelves, it contains a minimum amount of mold and bacteria. So yes, you've made some great progress.

But even the best all-natural foods may have some all-natural contaminants on them. Because you're eating veggies, beans, nuts, and fruits week after week, you need to have them as clean and allergen free as possible. Simply put, *washing with water is important, but it's not enough*!

There is an easy and cost-effective way to clean and take care of your food: Buy vitamin C crystals or powder, and use the mix I'm about to describe to clean your produce (veggies and fruits) as soon as you bring it home from the grocery store. Buy straight ascorbic acid powder only. Do not get ester C or buffered C.

Here's the process:

- First, run your organic greens and vegetables under fresh water, and wash off all the visible dirt and pollen.
- Pick out all wilted leaves and cut off all parts that are not edible.
- Fill a large glass bowl (one that holds at least a gallon of water) with water and add one heaping teaspoon of vitamin C crystals. Then soak those veggies and fruits without peels, such as berries and grapes, for ten to fifteen minutes. Use a separate bowl to soak greens, such as arugula and

spinach. This speeds up the process of rinsing and drying, plus it prevents cross-contamination of dirt and bugs. For dried beans, nuts, brown rice, and quinoa, soak only the amount to be cooked that day; the rest of the dried beans, grains, and seeds can be stored in a glass container in your pantry for future meals.

- Be sure to rinse well before eating or cooking.
- If you don't have one already, a salad spinner is a great household tool. Spin all the excess water out of your greens and fruit, and store them in a glass container with a sealed top.
- One final tip: Lay a small sheet of paper towel on top of the greens and fruit to absorb any excess moisture. Less moisture means less mold and bacterial growth.

As for the nuts, you can air-dry them or just pop them into the oven at 300°F. For a tasty snack, lightly coat the nuts with olive oil and sprinkle on dried herbs such as rosemary. Yum.

Is this voodoo science? Not at all. Vitamin C (aka ascorbic acid) works because it kills the bacteria and fungi on your produce without harming *you*. Produce grown close to the earth will naturally have some of these microorganisms, and it's best to eliminate them altogether. Ascorbic acid also prevents oxidation, which helps your fruits and veggies stay fresher throughout the week. So when you bite into those carrots, you'll hear a crisp crunch instead of a soggy snap. For the same reason, if you add fresh lime juice (containing lots of natural vitamin C) to a slice of avocado, it will not turn brown for hours.

So I'll bet you think you have to go on an obscure Swedish health website to find these magical crystals. Guess again. Vitamin C crystals (sometimes labeled as vitamin C powder) are available at any health food store. They should come with a warning label: "Molds and bacteria, beware!"

Action item. Buy vitamin C powder or crystals and wash all your fruits, nuts, beans, and veggies in a solution of vitamin C and filtered water.

Step 3: Upgrade Your Kitchenware

Depending on what your pots and pans are made of, small amounts of metallic or chemical residue may be leaching into your food. Metals and toxins from kitchenware can easily build up in your system, damaging the helpful bioflora in the gut and generating digestive sensitivities. The ingestion of metals such as aluminum and nickel (from stainless steel) can also cause rashes, hives, and low energy. Beyond these allergic symptoms, the ingestion of metals and toxic coatings may also put undue stress on your liver, kidneys, and other vital organs, including your brain and heart.

If we're going to start by eliminating one type of pan, it should be the nonstick pans coated with PFOA that we talked about at the beginning of this chapter. As you will recall, occupational studies show that the PFOA in nonstick coating can be carcinogenic and is not recommended for human ingestion. It may decrease energy and mental concentration in the short term and burden your system in the long term.

Stainless-steel cookware is widely available and a popular choice for many. But let's not forget, it contains nickel and other metals that can leach into your best stir-fry veggies. Stainless-steel kettles may infuse your hot water with extra nickel as well—not something you want to drink. Nickel gives many people, including my son, contact dermatitis. But if ingested, it can cause symptoms such as nausea, diarrhea, and vomiting, and if inhaled, it can cause severe damage to the lungs and kidneys.[8] Like many metals such as arsenic and mercury, nickel isn't easily processed and detoxified by the body, so it accumulates in tissues and organs. Avoiding it is the best policy.

Aluminum pots and pans are less expensive than some others, but that may be their only advantage. Although aluminum is the third most abundant element in the earth's crust, it is not known to be of any benefit to the human body and biochemistry. Like nickel, aluminum can cause contact dermatitis and, if ingested, can cause digestive and kidney disorders. There are also some studies showing that at high levels, it may be linked to breast cancer[9] (possibly from exposure to underarm deodorant) and even Alzheimer's disease.[10]

So does this mean you should stop using aluminum foil? Sorry to say, yes! Convenient as it is, it has all the same problems that come from pots and pans with toxic metals in them. Acidic and salty foods react with aluminum and may even cause more harmful substances to leach into your dish, so be sure to avoid cooking with these metal pans and pots at all costs.

At a more general level, pots and pans with plastic handles pose a big risk because these can emit toxic fumes if heated. Best to bid them a tearful good-bye and good riddance. And if you have *any* of these types of pots that are worn, chipped, or cracked, I recommend that you discard them immediately.

So now that I've turned your whole kitchen upside down, I want you to know that there is definitely a bright side. You may be jettisoning some kitchenware, but you'll be gaining a whole new level of allergy health. Once you feel the effects, you'll know that saying farewell to that twelve-year-old nonstick pan was well worth it.

The transition to allergy-friendly kitchenware probably won't happen overnight. But I'm hoping you'll be inspired to get rid of some of the more *problematic* items immediately and build up your collection of healthful kitchenware as soon as you can.

The best pots and pans to use are *glass*, *enamel*, and *cast iron*. These are not always the cheapest, but many of them can be bought for around the same cost as your average stainless-steel set. Glass is mainly silica—basically sand—and does not present any dangers to your health. Look for glass pots and pans that are made with sodium borosilicate glass (Pyrex is one brand). It has relatively low coefficients of thermal expansion, making it more durable than most glass and less vulnerable to thermal shock. Glass holds up extremely well under heat, so its biggest vulnerability probably has more to do with being dropped than being used for cooking. I love using my German-made glass teakettle I found in a shop in Koreatown, Los Angeles.

> The best pots and pans to use are *glass*, *enamel*, and *cast iron*.

Cast iron is one of my favorite kitchenware materials. I have one pan that has been in my family for thirty-five years! If the iron pan or pot is well maintained, food won't stick, and you won't need to use soap, as you usually must on other cookware. Just scrub with warm water and keep it seasoned with oil. And if blood tests have indicated that you have low iron levels, using a cast-iron pan can actually be helpful by supplementing the daily iron requirements. Iron is one mineral that is essential to our energy, bones, and red blood cells. Menstruating women often are iron anemic due to monthly loss of blood, and using cast-iron pots and pans can supplement their deficiencies. You will slowly ingest more iron over time just by cooking with this kind of skillet, especially if you cook acidic foods such as tomato sauce. I have an iron wok and use it to cook my dairy-free Bolognese sauce and stir-fry vegetables.

Green cookware is a new entry to the market and has a big upside. It's made with either stainless-steel or aluminum that has been coated heavily with nonstick ceramic that's free of PFOA-contaminated material. Some people find that after a few uses, these pans can lose some of that nonstick quality, but if you take good care of your cookware and get a high-quality ceramic product, it's wonderfully convenient for omelets and other sticky foods.

All-ceramic or clay pots and pans have been used for centuries and are still very popular in many parts of the world. Look online for reputable companies that make lead-free, unglazed, non-varnished clay pots. With little or no oil, you can steam your vegetables, slow-cook your beans, make soups, and cook meats and poultry.

If you like to bake gluten-free delights, clayware is also fun to use. It needs some care in handling due to its fragile nature, and some items can be more porous than others and thus absorb chemicals more easily. Follow directions on how to use and wash these items. I found my 100 percent ceramic large pots at the local Korean grocery store, and I use them regularly for soups, stews, and steaming vegetables. I even use it to make my Korean brown rice porridge with sesame oil! I am happy they aren't too expensive. (I've broken a few already.)

Pizza stones are a great alternative to metal baking sheets. Look for the ones made from clay or ceramic. Please, do not use anything made from natural granite. We love our kitchens to be beautifully designed and functional, and granite is lovely, durable, and easy to wipe off. There's just one problem; it can naturally contain toxic metals such as arsenic, mercury, and lead, and radioactive elements such as uranium, thallium, and plutonium (yes, plutonium!). So best not to lick off any food that falls on your countertop—especially acidic foods such as your favorite marinara sauce.

Bamboo steamers are as all natural as you can get and are a great way to cook vegetables while preserving much of their nutritional content.

Instead of aluminum foil, try unbleached, chlorine-free parchment paper (found in health food stores). Often used in baking, it can withstand the same high temperatures that aluminum foil can—up to 425ºF—but without the disadvantages. I even use it in place of plastic sandwich bags whenever I need to take my scrumptious veggie-laden, gluten-free sandwich on the run.

Who doesn't love barbecued corn on the cob? "Wrap in aluminum foil" is in pretty much every recipe on how to make the best barbecued corn. If the natural corn husk (always my first choice) isn't available, I use parchment paper instead! It's quite easy—all you need is the parchment paper, clarified butter (ghee), salt, and organic corn. Rub the butter evenly on the corn, lightly salt, and roll everything up in parchment paper, and twist the ends tightly. Place it on the top shelf of the grill, so it doesn't cook directly over the fire. It may take twenty-five to forty minutes, depending on your grill temperature, but the results will be the most amazing corn you ever tasted! Don't fret if the ends of the paper get a little singed—it's much better than aluminum, and the corn inside will be delicious!

You can do the same to bake sweet potatoes, steam fish, or cook anything else that normally requires aluminum foil. It's biodegradable, and it's better for your allergies and better for the environment! Just be sure not to go above 425ºF, otherwise the paper may burst into flames.

Another great alternative to foil and plastic wraps for covering bowls and pots for food storage are reusable silicone lids, such as those made in Italy. Colorful silicone kitchen implements and bakeware have been popping up everywhere. Silicone is a synthetic material made of bonded silica (sand) and oxygen. I have researched the safety aspect of these products extensively, and so far, they are considered safe and made of inert material that will not leach out any chemicals, even if you use them at high heat (up to 428ºF). I have now replaced my plastic ice trays with silicone ones shaped like starfish and seashells.

Now, one more tip, especially if you get itchy skin rashes or hives. You've purified your kitchen of nonstick pans, aluminum, and stainless steel. But what about your utensils—spatulas, tongs, ladles, and all the rest? Are they made of stainless steel, brass, or aluminum? Some metals, such as the nickel in stainless steel and the copper in brass, may be the root cause of your allergic reaction. Plastic utensils are not any better, because they have their own problems. The European Union Commission has banned plastics containing BPA altogether. I hope this will also happen in the United States soon.

Wooden or bamboo utensils (available at any health food store with kitchenware) are terrific, and so are ceramic porcelain spoons (found in Asian markets). Wooden chopsticks are one of my favorites because they force me to slow down and be more present with my eating. My food seems to taste better when I take the time and care to eat it with chopsticks. And I can even use one to keep my hair from falling in my face while cooking!

Action item. Get glass, enamel, or cast-iron pots and pans; wooden utensils; porcelain spoons; and wooden chopsticks.

Step 4: Go Plastic Free

It's hard to think of any substance that can be molded into as many shapes and sizes as plastic or that can be used in everything from toys to sandwich containers to bubble wrap. There are at least three good reasons why plastic became so popular over the past half century: convenience, durability, and cost. And with the promise of widespread three-dimensional printing on the horizon, the ubiquity of plastic seems assured for the foreseeable future.

But as I explained at the beginning of this chapter, plastics are harmful to you and your children, and they can leach into our food when we eat from them, microwave in them, and store food in them. Plastic toys and baby bottles can be detrimental to your child's health. Children quickly absorb the chemicals released by plastics, and a child's small body weight and frame means that the toxins will cause more cellular damage and immunological issues than in someone three to six times as large. Endocrine-disrupting, brain-fogging, hive- and rash-producing plastics should be banned from your kitchen.

The good news is post-plastic life in the kitchen is not as hard as it sounds. Remember, humans got along just fine without it for over 99.9 percent of their existence on earth. Even a three-quarters reduction in your use of plastic can work wonders. And if those low-energy days start to become a thing of the past and all the itching and other allergic symptoms recede, who's going to insist that they still need plastic?

1. **STORAGE WARE.** Most of us have some kind of plastic storage ware in our homes. It's so convenient, so well marketed, and so cheap that almost every household in America has some. I grew up using it, but now that I know about the harmful health effects of plastics, I've made sure my child won't grow up doing the same. All plastics have the potential to leach into our food, especially if they are heated or used to store acidic foods such as tomato sauce or citrus juice. But allergy-free health requires some deep changes, and our overreliance on plastic is one of those things we must question. I can't tell you how many patients I've seen who needed a little "plastic surgery" for their energy level and concentration to start picking back up again.

While I favor using fresh foods whenever possible, I know that our busy lives make storing leftovers a necessity. But instead of standard plastic storage ware, get glass containers, which are much better for both food preservation and your overall health.

Just as with your pots and pans, glass is preferable to other materials, which can easily emit toxic and allergenic metals or synthetic chemicals. If you have leftovers in the fridge, I recommend freezing part of it to prevent spoiling and to give you more variety to choose from. Freezing will prevent bacteria and mold overgrowth, and you can simply reheat your delicious dish a few days later. As we talked about in step 1, don't let those veggies wilt away in the fridge, then eat them five days later. Keep them stored in glass, and then freeze what you can't immediately consume within a couple of days. Remember to cool your hot leftovers to room temperature before storing them in glass to prevent the container from cracking. Also, when removing a glass container from the freezer, allow the food to thaw at room temperature; putting it under hot water can also crack the glass.

For this reason—and because I have a perpetually hungry family—I have a freezer in the garage, entirely separate from my refrigerator. This way, I'm never out of food and I'm not trying to jam-pack a tiny icebox with weeks' worth of lentil soup and collard greens. I label each glass container with a sticky note saying what's stored inside and the date it was frozen. Then, when I'm pressed and don't have time to prepare dinner; I pull out the dish that has been in the freezer the longest, usually under a month. Whenever I cook, I make large quantities of soup, pasta sauce, grilled chicken, and beans so I always have something to pull out at the last minute.

To avoid storing your food in plastic, I recommend immediately transferring any packaged goods—brown rice, gluten-free oats, beans, nuts, and seeds—into glass containers. The reason is that anything sitting in a package is prone to mold, especially if it has already been opened. Move the bag of chips into a glass container. And from now on, every time you unload from the grocery store, begin your food transference ritual right then: Everything out of plastic, into glass. After a few weeks of practice, this will become routine.

2. TEAPOTS. Some people like to use electric teapots for the convenience. Plastic alert! Although the water is heated inside a metal casing, the outside of the teapot is usually made of a plastic that can emit BPA and other chemicals. When the BPA leaches into your water, you're drinking a BPA-infused hot drink. Better to use a covered glass pot or an enamel kettle to boil your purified water. It's also better for energy consumption because a lot of us leave our appliances plugged in all day. Donate or recycle your electric teapot instead. And as we discussed earlier, glass stovetop kettles beat out metal ones any day.

3. CUTTING BOARDS. Many of my patients think that wooden cutting boards are more attractive to bacteria and mold than their synthetic counterparts. Not true. I heartily recommend a wooden cutting board, which, if taken care of properly, is no more germophilic than a plastic one. Chopping on plastic is an ideal way to have toxic particles trickle into your food. Chop on wood, on the other hand, and you're not even likely to get a splinter.

Just be sure to clean your cutting board with all-natural soap and hot running water regularly, and you'll be fine. Glass or ceramic boards are also available and work fine; just be careful in handling them. Also, never wash your wooden cutting boards—or anything else wooden—in the automatic dishwasher. This dries out the wood and leads to a higher incidence of cracking.

4. KITCHEN UTENSILS. By now you know the drill. If you're sautéing and frying with a plastic spatula, go back to a nice wooden one or maybe bamboo. Lots of frying pans have plastic handles that, if accidentally heated, can emit toxic gases. Again, if you make the switch to glass, cast iron, or enamel, this shouldn't be a problem.

Lots of children have plastic sippy cups, but these can leach phthalates or BPA into their drinks, especially if the juice is squeezed from acidic fruits such as oranges or pineapples. Look for children's cups with labels saying they are free of BPA and phthalates. Plenty of water bottles and cups are made of glass or porcelain. Reusing plastic forks may be of some minor benefit to the environment, but it's bad for your health. Recycle them, and get a reusable bamboo spoon, fork, knife, and chopstick set that comes with a fabric holder available at most health food stores. I carry a set in my purse and use them when appropriate (not at five-star establishments!), at restaurants that only provide plastic utensils. To prevent soiling my purse, I rinse them in the restroom after every use.

Action item. Eliminate all plastics in the kitchen. Buy a glass teapot and storage containers and wooden cutting boards. Store all packaged goods in glass containers. Recycle all plastic utensils, spatulas, cups, and pans with plastic handles.

Step 5: Get Control of Your Electronic Appliances

1. MICROWAVE OVEN. Every home has one, but not every home *needs* one. I hope someday the microwave will go the way of the VHS cassette and the eight-track tape: good for nostalgia value but not much else.

Sure, microwaves heat food quickly. Back in the early 1980s, we felt a certain sense of futuristic magic from popping a frozen chicken pot pie in and watching it come out bubbling and sizzling only minutes later. And over time, we've grown to expect such convenience as a matter of course. But when it comes to your health in the twenty-first century, there is much to be concerned about with microwaves.

Microwaving foods exposes them to electromagnetic radiation and results in a change in their polarity (positive and negative charge) up to a million times a second. Water is particularly susceptible to these changes in polarity. The result is that microwaved molecules are denatured (chemical bonds broken), and the nutritional value of microwaved food is much reduced.

One well-known example of the negative effects of microwave use is that of human breast milk. Normal human breast milk has bacteria-fighting enzymes called lysozymes, and microwaving tends to destroy these. The result is increased bacterial growth in microwaved milk, making babies more likely to catch diseases. "Even at 20°C to 25°C, *E. coli* growth was five times that of control human milk. Microwaving appears to be contraindicated at high temperatures, and questions regarding its safety exist even at low temperatures."[11]

We all know that microwave ovens emit radiation, but it is not well contained within those four flimsy walls. If you are ever around a microwave, stand at least five feet away while it is running. Better yet, stop using it altogether.

2. TOASTERS. Toasters and toaster ovens use a lot of electricity to heat your leftovers or toast that tasty gluten-free, yeast-free bread. Remember how we want all electrical appliances turned off at nighttime? That's because electromagnetic radiation can be disruptive to normal cell function, and toasters are one of the most power-packed forms of electromagnetic energy in the home. When using your toaster, stay away from it while it heats up your food. When it's not in use, unplug it! This includes all the other kitchen appliances, such as coffeemaker, blender, electric can opener, and all the rest. You'll be saving energy in the process.

> When it's not in use, unplug it!

Action item. Stop using the microwave and use the toaster oven instead to heat up leftovers. And whatever electric appliance you use, stand far away from it while it's running. By the way, gas stove tops do not generate much electricity, so you can cook over them for hours without worrying about the electromagnetic factor!

By now you have vastly reduced the number of the most common allergens in your life. By cleaning your external environment, improving the quality of your air and water, eating an allergy-free diet, and clearing out and cleaning up your living areas, you have knocked a huge dent in your toxic load. So take some time to congratulate yourself and realize that what you're doing isn't always easy. As you go forward, be sure to *clarify your intention.* What I mean by this is simply to remember what drove you to commit to living an allergy-free life. Remember what you struggled with *before* you dedicated yourself to this program and envision the kind of life you want to live *after* your allergies fade away into distant memory. Instead of the day-to-day grind, see the big picture: Your new life without allergies!

DAY 6

CLEAN UP YOUR
BODY

For these final two days of our weeklong journey to renewed allergy health, we're going to pay special attention to the allergens you expose yourself to at the most intimate levels: your *body* and your *emotions*. We all have heard about the intimate link between the body and mind. Psychosomatic connections are no longer accepted only by people into alternative health and wellness—now they are considered mainstream science. Simply put, the state of your body affects your emotions, and vice versa. Your emotional and psychological resilience can help your body heal.

That's why I am convinced that as you recover from your allergy symptoms, you will find new emotions cropping up. A healed body also feels more vibrant. Over time, these new thoughts and feelings will give you messages about what you hope to reconnect with now that your body can process allergic reactions better. You may find a new desire presenting itself—for instance, a new urge to spend more time outside in nature. You may remember a project or two you left by the wayside when allergies were holding you back. But, of course, life after allergies isn't always fun and games. I know from experience that the more your allergies recede, the more you'll be able to deal with difficult emotions as well. A body no longer at war with itself has more space to handle the emotional turmoil of our stressful lives. And as you heal some of the emotional scars from having lived with allergies for so long, your body will return to its calm and healthy natural state. Sympathetic dominance and a life lived in a fight, fright, or flight mode caused by allergens will transform into an abiding sense of physical relaxation and well-being. And if you happen to inhale a stray mold spore or a little pollen falls on your eyelids, your body will have a much easier time dealing with it.

I'm sure that's part of why you bought this book in the first place. You know that only by healing your allergies will you be able to get back the emotional clarity and focus you need to do what you were meant to do in life. With allergies, life revolves around *fighting the body*. Without allergies, life revolves around *fulfilling your purpose*. When the body is in its optimal healthy state, a different psychological space can open up. You aren't running to doctors or stocking up on antihistamines as if the world were about to end. You don't feel sluggish and run-down anymore. Your eyes are no longer the same color as those organic beets you're now eating, and you're not closing in on the world record for sneezes per minute. My hope is that soon the emotional agony of those grueling months and years you've spent will start to fade away. The despair, frustration, and powerlessness will start to become a thing of the past.

If there's one "ailment" that nearly all my patients have in common when I meet them, it's that they rarely take enough time to nurture and heal their bodies. I tell them, "It's not your fault; it's part of American culture." Think about it. We're stuck in traffic every morning and evening, and we eat lunch at our desks during ten- or twelve-hour workdays. By the time we make it home, we often have barely enough energy to make dinner and help the kids with homework before we fall asleep. Time for exercise? Oh, if only! I know it's tough to get those thirty minutes in three or four times a week. But you'd be dazzled by the healthful effects of exercise on your allergies. We'll talk a bit more about them in a few pages.

Yet not all the blame can fall on our culture or stressful workdays. Too many of us put family, friends, and obligations ahead of *ourselves* and *our* physical well-being. What's easier to justify: helping your spouse around the house or checking out for an hour at the spa? I want to tell you something vitally important: You deserve time for your body. Not only do you deserve it but I'm *mandating* it as part of your allergy makeover! That means yes to baths, to spas, to massages, and to time for relaxation and breathing. You simply can't have optimal allergy health without making the proper care of your body a part of your life. But a focus on your body also means exercise (although, as you'll see, this doesn't mean you must turn into a gym rat or become a Pilates expert). Finally, we'll have to reduce the toxic load in your hygiene and beauty products so that eyeliner doesn't become yet another allergy threat.

Why is it so important to take care of your body in this way? It all starts with the skin. The skin is the largest organ in the body and probably also the most neglected. Some people call it the "third lung" because it breathes, in the sense that substances can exit through the pores (via sweat) and enter through them as well (for example, when you take a shower in chlorinated water). The skin forms a semipermeable barrier against the external world and works to regulate your temperature, communicate with the external environment through proprioceptive organs (touch, pain, pressure), and excrete metabolic waste and toxins. Be thankful for all the work it does! However, for these reasons, the skin is *highly* susceptible to allergens and demands extra attention. If an allergen doesn't make it into your body by way of your food, air, or water, there's a good chance it will find a way in through your skin. Properly caring for our skin is probably something we all could stand to learn a bit more about.

WHAT'S IN *YOUR* MAKEUP?

Before we jump into the new body makeover, let's look at some of the chemicals you're likely to find in your beauty and hygiene products, so you know exactly what you might be exposing yourself to.

Amines

Watch out for anything containing amines such as diethanolamine, triethanolamine, and monoethanolamine. They're used in beauty products to balance pH, help with foaming, and preserve the product. But one thing they *won't* help preserve is your health. That's because amines, when mixed with nitrates, can form compounds that are carcinogenic. But their day-to-day effects can be just as irritating. Many of my patients have reported skin irritations and even dermatitis that we linked back to the use of amine-containing cosmetics.

Phthalates

Funny spelling aside, phthalates are nothing to laugh at. They're often used as lubricants but can also show up in perfume, nail polish, and a host of beauty products. Phthalates are known endocrine disruptors, leading California to place a ban on using them in children's toys, effective in 2009. Their negative effect on proper childhood development is clear evidence that we shouldn't be using them. Both PBS and *60 Minutes* have aired specials covering the case against phthalates, and these are online for you to watch. While phthalates' potential effects on adults are the subject of some controversy, there's no reason not to eliminate them during your makeup makeover.

Sodium Lauryl Sulfate

Sodium lauryl sulfate (SLS) is an ingredient used for foaming, most often in soaps and shampoos. (Sodium laureth sulfate is basically the same thing.) While you might get a few extra suds out of it, you're also opening yourself to the organ damage, neurotoxicity, and carcinogenic effects that SLS brings with it. Anything that contributes to your toxic load puts one more hurdle between you and allergy relief. Remember, the closer these chemicals get to your skin and face, the more likely they are to find their way into your system.

Mercury

Mercury? *In cosmetics?* Say it ain't so! Yes, it's sad but true; that chemical we strive to avoid by eating less tuna and swordfish is in many of our cosmetics. Besides being a poison in large doses, mercury exposure can cause anxiety, changes in sight, memory issues, numbness in the hands and feet, and irritability. Even though banned for use in cosmetics in this country, mercury finds its way into these products from overseas. The most frequent sources of mercury are cosmetics aimed at face and skin care, especially in antiaging and skin-lightening products. The FDA website urges "consumers not to use skin creams, beauty and antiseptic soaps, or lotions that might contain mercury," many of which are sold illegally in the United States.[1] Anything without a label showing its ingredients, especially if you suspect it is foreign-made, should not be used for skin care purposes.

But even the *vapors* from products containing mercury can expose us to their harmful effects unawares. Check to make sure your family members are not using these products unknowingly, so you are not breathing them in. The FDA urges you to discard anything that has mercury or mercurous chloride, or calomel; the word *mercuric*; or any mercury compound listed on the package.[2]

Step 1: Get a Makeup-Free Makeover

At what age did you first use makeup? Twelve? Eleven? Younger? You can probably still remember the pride you got in feeling more adult, more like a real woman. The foundation and blush went on, then the lipstick, and there you were, a full-fledged adult (or almost). By the time we really grow up, many of us have been using makeup for *decades* without once stopping to examine just what we were putting on our skin.

In working out our cosmetic routines, I think we need to consider the facts carefully. If you are suffering from allergies, I want you to consider this section very carefully when you make your decisions about your daily beauty ritual. The face and especially the lips and eyes are very vulnerable parts of your body, having less of a natural barrier than other areas. When you apply makeup to these areas, there is a higher absorption rate than if you applied the same chemicals elsewhere.

And what's in makeup? Potentially, three of the things we talked about earlier in this chapter: sodium lauryl sulfate, amines, and phthalates. But makeup can also have harmful VOCs

(chemicals that are partly responsible for smog), such as formaldehyde, and other toxins that no one should be exposed to so directly.
Studies show that toxic metals such as lead and mercury can be
found in lipsticks and facial creams. Nail polish is loaded with
VOCs and is a real concentration and energy disruptor. Here is a
list of some of the very *worst* chemicals in personal products,
known endocrine disruptors and possible carcinogens as well:
formaldehyde, benzene, toluene, ethylbenzene, acetone, methac-
rylates, and cyclohexane. Check the back of each beauty product
to see if you are being exposed to these chemicals, other VOCs,
sodium lauryl sulfate, amines, or phthalates, and get rid of them
first. If the ingredients are not listed on the bottle or container
(which they legally should be) or have worn off from use, go online
and look them up. You'll usually be able to find a complete list of
ingredients on the manufacturer's website.

So what to do now that half your cosmetic stash is gone? I
know that for personal or professional reasons, getting rid of *all*
makeup can be tough. When looking at the remaining half, which
is still full of synthetic chemicals, consider the risks you are taking
with your skin and how much these toxins may be exacerbating
your allergy symptoms. Get rid of everything you possibly can. But
if, for whatever reason, you feel the need to hold on to a few of your
cosmetics, try to reduce your dependence on them. Can you go
from wearing lipstick seven days a week to just five or even three?
Can you skip the eyeliner or mascara for one night? Can you go a
day or two a week makeup free altogether? Work your way up to
seven-day makeup-free living one day at a time.

There's also another alternative. Try all-natural makeup products instead. Many websites will have makeup made entirely of
plant-based ingredients that do not harm the skin. However, even
some kinds of makeup that appear to be green may actually contain some of the chemicals we've talked about in this chapter, so

read the labels carefully. Anything with synthetic fragrances or with preservatives is almost a surefire bet for toxins.

Don't worry, though. There's good news for those of you who love to look fresh and fabulous. What I've found is that by follow-

Dalia came into my office with numbness on her tongue and lips. She was fifty-five years old, married with two children in college, and had very little stress in her life. The numbness started in her tongue first, then spread to her lips. It was constant, and she worried that she was losing her sense of taste. Kissing her husband was not the same anymore. She could move her lips and tongue, but she couldn't feel them, as if she had gotten a shot of Novocain. She went to her internist, who had no answers and referred her to a neurologist, but still she was no closer to a solution. It was getting worse, and by the time she came to see me, she had had the numbness symptoms for three months. After doing a detailed history and evaluation, I ordered a hair and urine analysis for heavy-metal toxins. Both tests indicated that she had high levels of lead. I asked her what type of lipstick, creams, and products she used on her skin and lips. It turned out that the new lipstick she had started using five months ago was on the FDA's list for high lead levels. She used it daily and reapplied it three to four times throughout the day—even more if she had a dinner party to go to. She also licked her lips frequently, which might explain why her tongue was numb too. Immediately, I asked her to stop applying all lipsticks and gave her some supplements to help her gently cleanse the lead out of her body and rebuild the affected nerves in her lips and tongue. Within four weeks, the numbness in Dalia's lips and tongue completely disappeared, and she was elated that the "anesthetic" had finally worn off.

ing the allergy-free dietary protocol laid out in Day 1, most of my patients have developed healthier and more vibrant-looking skin naturally.

1. SHAVING CREAM (FOR FACE OR BODY). Have you ever wondered what kinds of ingredients make up the average shaving cream? Most of shaving cream—up to 80 percent—is water, but unfortunately, some of the other ingredients may cause allergic reactions. For instance, triethanolamine (TEA) is a thickener, an emulsifying agent that keeps the water and oil from separating. The problem is it can cause contact dermatitis, and some formulas with TEA can be contaminated with nitrosamines, which have been linked to cancer. Another scary fact is that it is on the precursor list to making nitrogen mustard gas.[3]

Another suspicious ingredient is propylene glycol, a lubricant and humectant commonly found in antifreeze and brake fluid. It can be a skin irritant and is linked to allergies, immune toxicity, endocrine disruption, and even cancer. Propylene glycol is also used in many other different body care products such as shampoo, conditioner, soap, moisturizers, and toothpaste.

Definitely read your labels and look for nontoxic shaving creams or gels that contain natural ingredients free of chemicals. Here's a partial list:

- Natural moisturizers such as jojoba, coconut, shea butter, and macadamia and olive oils
- Aloe vera gel, which is soothing and healing for the skin
- Chamomile, a skin calmer and natural anti-inflammatory herb
- Calendula, which heals minor cuts and burns
- Evening primrose oil, which reduces itching and inflammation

2. PERSONAL AND INTIMACY LUBRICANTS. Many of my patients (both men and women) use a personal lubricant to enhance sensation and reduce friction and irritation during sex. Also women who have gone through menopause often complain of vaginal dryness and pain during intercourse, and lubricants can definitely help ease the discomfort and bring pleasure back into their sexual life. As with shaving cream, the number one ingredient is water, but the following chemicals sometimes found in lubricants are much less benign: glycerin (can promote yeast and bacterial infections), propylene glycol (skin irritant and possible endocrine disrupter), and methyl- and propylparaben (preservatives that are known carcinogens). These chemicals do not belong on or in your sensitive areas. Genital tissues are highly vascular and very thin skinned, so that much of the toxins can be readily absorbed in seconds.

Ten years ago, there were maybe two or three brands of personal lubricants, but now you may be able to find online many much healthier brands that are made from organic ingredients and are free of toxic chemicals and preservatives. There are three types of lubricants: water-, oil-, and silicone-based. I highly recommend that you try the all-natural water- and oil-based lubricants. Stay away from the synthetic silicone-based lubricants (which also can deteriorate latex condoms during intercourse).

Ladies, please take your own organic, all-natural lubricant and give it to your doctor to use in your annual gynecological exam. Wouldn't it be amazing if your doctor switched over to using the more healthful version!

A side note while we're on the subject of sexual health: latex condoms can cause allergic reactions and can be very drying and irritating to vaginal and penile skin. If you and your partner are free from viral infections such as human papillomavirus (HPV) and herpes and other sexually transmitted diseases (STDs), look for natural-skin condoms. Other nonlatex condoms are made of polyisoprene (a synthetic version of latex that is supposedly allergy free) and polyurethane (a synthetic condom that is latex free but stiffer and less stretchable).

Action item. Throw away all makeup containing toxic chemicals or minimize your use of them. Buy all-natural makeup if you need a replacement.

Step 2: Approach Hygiene the Natural Way

There's a deep corporeal reason that a shower is so appealing. Hot water refreshes the skin and revitalizes you like almost nothing else. It gets the blood flowing and your energy circulating. When you take care of your skin, your immunity is stronger because you aren't struggling with rashes, dirt, fungus, and bacteria. It also rinses away the pollen, smog, and industrial chemicals that can land on your skin during the day So yes, cleaning yourself *properly* is going to become part of our new allergy makeover. After all, if you want to wipe off traces of all kinds of household and environmental allergens, what could be better than a refreshing, hot shower?

I highly recommend a shower a day if you want to keep the allergy doctor away. Showering at night is preferable because you can rid yourself of everything that has built up on your skin during the course of the day. That way, you don't drag little pollen reminders of your afternoon walk onto your sheets and pillows. But if, for whatever reason, you can't take a shower at night, at least clean your feet because there is nowhere else on the body that fungus and bacteria can build up so quickly. Do you *really* want to cover your feet all day in a pair of sweaty socks and then put them straight into those clean sheets?

Whether it's a foot washing or a long shower to wipe away the dirt, smog, pollen, and other allergens, you don't need to roll out a set of high-tech synthetic compounds to get clean. Mother Nature has plenty of ways to cleanse, exfoliate, and moisturize without ever using a chemical laboratory. Our principle of buying only all-natural, chemical- and preservative-free products makes choosing easy. We're lucky that most health food stores and even some of the national drugstore chains carry all-natural alternatives for some things, such as toothpaste and deodorant. Even the big-box super-stores have begun to catch on to the fundamental importance of going all natural with beauty and hygiene products. Let's hope their foresight continues.

So next time you hit the shower, here's how to protect your skin in the most allergy-friendly way possible:

1. **SOAP.** There are oatmeal, avocado, and lavender soaps, and honey, juniper, peppermint, and vanilla soaps. Sometimes soaps can sound more like the beginnings of a recipe than something to wash your body with. Nothing is better for your skin than these plant-based soaps with their natural cleansing power.

This bit of wisdom comes with a big caveat, though. If you buy a vanilla soap, you want it to have real vanilla and *only* real plant products. No pentaerythrityl tetra-di-*t*-butyl hydroxyhydrocinnamate (anything with that many letters is most likely a synthetic chemical), no D&C (U.S.-approved drug and cosmetics) yellow 7. Ingredient lists should read more like this: organic olive oil, organic lavender oil, organic coconut oil. See? All pronounceable words. Notice the difference? To decipher the ingredients of the first list, you would need a chemical dictionary, whereas everything on the second list might be growing in your backyard. (That would be an amazing backyard too!) Artificial fragrances and colors do not improve the cleansing action of the soap, and they can be irritating to your skin.

When you buy soap, think *mild, probiotic* soap. Probiotic foods such as sauerkraut, kimchi, miso soup, and, yes, even dark chocolate have become increasingly recognized for their health benefits and their ability to add helpful bacteria to the digestive system. (Remember, while yogurt made with cow's or goat's milk is also a probiotic food, you should avoid it if you have a dairy allergy. There are, however, delicious coconut and rice yogurts you can enjoy.) Probiotic soap adds helpful bioflora (good bacteria) to your hands and skin on top of removing dirt and the day's detritus.

You want a certain amount of healthful bacteria on your hands, which is why hand sanitizers and antibacterial soaps are to be avoided at all costs. They're *indiscriminate* bacteria killers. So although they may rid you of the "bad" bacteria, they also eliminate the bacteria that help stave off allergies and disease. Triclosan is the most common chemical used in antibacterial liquid hand soaps and dish-washing detergents. The toxic chemical has also been found to be in many other personal products, such as toothpaste, face wash, and deodorant, and in household items such as shower curtains, towels, mattresses, kitchenware, cutting boards, and even toys. Triclosan is linked to liver disorder and, at low levels, may even disrupt your thyroid function. It ends up in our water sources, lakes, rivers, and oceans because wastewater treatment does not remove it, and it can be very toxic to aquatic life. Watch out for labels that say "antibacterial," "protects against mold and mildew growth," "combats germs," "keeps food fresher," "eliminates odor." Try using just plain soap with hot water. According to the FDA advisory committee, it will do the same job in eliminating bacteria and other microbes.

And when you squirt yourself with that sanitizer, you'll also be inundated with a host of synthetic chemicals. Hand sanitizers do not prevent hand-to-mouth contamination, and the chemicals can be adsorbed straight into your body transdermally. Avoid it, *please*! Again, the best way to remove dirt, grease, and germs is with soap and hot water.

Even some seemingly all-natural soaps may have chemicals, so read the labels carefully. To set your mind at ease, you might want to buy your soaps online from an all-natural beauty products store. Soaps that seem to be naturally scented may sound (and smell) good, but in practice, they can have synthetically made scents that cause allergic reactions—irritating your eyes and nose and even causing headaches.

2. SHAMPOO AND CONDITIONER. As with soap, use all-natural, unscented shampoos. Shampoos are especially likely to contain sodium lauryl sulfate (for foaming), which can be a strong skin irritant, causing dermatitis and rashes. Nonallergenic shampoos can be found at health food stores and even local convenience stores. Ordering online is also an option. I know from personal use that hair conditioners found in the health food stores do not work as well as commercial brands. Hair texture varies widely from one head to another. I have Korean hair, which is very coarse, and it's difficult to soften the strands with the organic conditioners. I found that a light hair oil such as argan oil or Moroccan oil added to the hair ends does a superb job of reducing hair flyaways and static. It will make your hair look healthy, with a vibrant sheen.

Most of us are tempted to skip shampooing for a few days so we can keep the beautiful hairdo that cost us a small fortune and half an afternoon at the stylist's. I know: "Just one of the small sacrifices we make for fashion," you say. And though it may help you keep that lovely style a few extra days, it also promotes bacterial and fungal growth on the scalp. I recommend that you shampoo every other day, if not every day. In the long run, your hair will be happier, and so will you.

Facial Eczema or Something Else?

Stacy, a young mother of two boys, worked full-time as a dental receptionist. She came into my office with a rash all around her hairline and forehead. Her doctor diagnosed her with eczema and prescribed a hydrocortisone cream and a special facial wash. After six weeks of diligently using the cream and wash, it seemed to be getting worse, so she decided to try alternative methods and get a second opinion. I took a closer look at her forehead and hairline and noticed a great deal of dandruff on her shoulders and even on the back of her sweater. Parting her hair, I took a closer look and found a severe case of fungal scalp infection. The skin on her forehead was not eczema—it was just an extension of the fungal infection on her scalp! No wonder the hydrocortisone cream didn't work! I asked her how often she washed her hair, and she said every seven to ten days. She complained that she was way too busy with work, spouse, and children to wash her hair. I told her that to heal her scalp, daily hair washing with a natural tea tree oil shampoo would be part of the treatment protocol. For her face and scalp, I also gave her an all-natural topical ointment that eradicates fungal infections. She came back a week later with at least 50 percent improvement of her skin condition *and* her dandruff. One month later, she came in with a big smile on her lovely, clear face, and beautiful flowing hair free of dandruff and fungi.

3. FACIAL AND SKIN CARE PRODUCTS. Remember, when it comes to heavy metals, toxins, and synthetics, your face is especially vulnerable. It's one area where I've found being especially careful with your product choices pays off big time. Fragrances, preservatives, dyes, and alcohols abound in facial and skin care

products. Moisturizers and lotions that come at this cost aren't worth it. Wrinkle and antiaging creams can be just as harmful, and let me just add a reminder to be on the lookout for those that might contain mercury (discussed earlier in this chapter).

New allergy-free skin care, along with exercise, is your new fountain of youth. As you follow the dietary tips and other allergy tips, your skin *will* look better than you ever thought it could. When you do buy skin care products, go organic as much as possible. Some plant-based products, despite being all natural, may react with your skin, so ask for samples first if you can. Test them on a patch of your skin to see if you get hives, rash, or any other allergic reaction.

4. DEODORANT. Here's one of my easy body care tips: to minimize bad odors, keep your underarm hair short. Longer hair that collects sweat encourages growth of yeast and bacteria, which are at the root of the not-so-good smells. By shaving and trimming it, you minimize the need for chemical smells to cover up, and if you wash with probiotic soap, body odor drops dramatically!

It's important not to use antiperspirants because these are chemical storehouses. A simple all-natural deodorant is enough to maintain a pleasant smell while allowing your body to sweat and excrete toxins through the pores naturally.

5. FOOT CARE. An all-natural way to treat your feet is to bathe them in warm water mixed with a touch of Himalayan or Dead Sea salt. These salts will help treat eczema, psoriasis, and fungi that grow on the feet. If you have fungal toenails, this mixture will help soften them and make them easier to clip away. Earlier, I said to be sure to wash your feet with soap and water before going to bed because they can be a breeding ground for bacteria and fungi, not to mention all the dirt and sweat accumulated from the day. Crawling into bed with unclean feet can promote fungal growth and skin disease. If you take a bath or a full-body shower before bed, even better.

Action item. Buy only all-natural and chemical- and preservative-free body care products. Look for probiotic soap for full body care and Dead Sea salts for nightly foot baths.

Step 3: Take a Bath

Bathing helps the blood circulate, increasing oxygenation to the cells. A good bath will also reduce inflammation and allow your skin to sweat out toxins that a simple shower can't. Reducing inflammation and toxins means fewer allergies. And everyone knows that a bath gives you a sense of calm that a yogi might envy. A bath makes your body less reactive to stressors in the environment, so that allergens can't bring down your day so easily. So why don't we bathe more often?

The truth is, many of us look at baths as a luxury. We get images of a candlelit bathroom, bubble bath, and maybe even champagne. Bathing seems like something for the idle rich, not for those of us who have to work, take care of kids, and manage a house. Bathing and rushing about from place to place are antonyms, or so it would seem. To bathe and enjoy it, you *do* need to relax, make time for yourself, and enjoy being in your body.

That's exactly what I want you to do starting today. Caring for your body is *not* a luxury any more. Taking care of your health and healing your allergies is not something you do in your spare time, whenever you can fit it in. Instead, think of it as a new focus to help bring back the vibrancy and energy you deserve to have. I want you to nourish your body, love it, and give it all the help you can so it can do its healing work. From now on, your bath will be a part of your allergy-healing program. If you can take a real, honest-to-goodness tub bath even once a week, the physical turnaround you experience can be dramatic. So let me share how to bathe for maximum allergy-relieving results.

THE BATHING PROCESS. First, prepare for the bath by buying a scrubbing mitt if you don't already have one. Also, get a bucket so you can douse yourself with water (explained later). Second, always take a shower *before* you bathe. Showering with probiotic soap will remove most of the dirt and toxins from your skin so you are not soaking in them while you bathe. When you shower, don't take a short, or military, shower. Spend time scrubbing everywhere, including your feet because harmful fungi and bacteria can take root there.

Third, when you take your bath, you want to soak in water that's hot but not too hot, so you don't unnecessarily shock the body. Spend about twenty to thirty minutes in the bathtub. This can also be a good time to take stock of how you've been feeling throughout the week and which of your allergy symptoms have popped up recently and which seem to be feeling better. It's an ideal opportunity for a weekly allergy makeover check-in with yourself. If something doesn't feel right, make note of it and see if you have changed anything about your diet or lifestyle. Did you eat a little more dairy or forget to run the air purifier? Did things get a little hectic this week, adding to your emotional stress? Check for correlations between the things that have changed in your lifestyle, and the allergy symptoms you might be feeling.

After the bath, with your body still wet, sit on a shower stool in the shower or tub. Use your scrubbing mitt to remove excess dead skin by scrubbing in a back-and-forth motion. You will see the layers of dead skin just peeling off. Be gentle on your skin because the scrubbing cloth can be quite abrasive. Turn the shower back on to fill the bucket with warm water, and splash the water on your arms, legs, and body to wash away dead skin, chemicals, and debris.

The splashing stimulation of your entire body will be invigorating and will improve your skin's integrity and elasticity, strengthen the immune and lymphatic systems, and even increase your metabolism. In fact, you may start sweating during the scrubbing process. Don't worry, it's normal. After you've done this a few times, your new skin will positively *glow* and feel as soft as a baby's.

Once your body-buzzing scrub down is complete, you can finish by washing your hair with an all-natural shampoo and slathering your body with one of those probiotic soaps I recommended. To keep your new skin moist and soft, apply an all-natural body cream or body butter. Now a tip to enhance your relaxation. If possible, after your bath ritual, *don't rush into any new activity.* Give your body time to adjust. The best thing to do is simply to lie down for ten to fifteen minutes so you can cool down and let your body return to its normal state and temperature. You'll notice a sense of calm and feelings of being connected to your body. You will also likely feel energized without any accompanying anxiety or nervousness. Who needs coffee now?

A weekly bath will greatly improve your body's ability to heal chronic allergies by sweating and detoxing unwanted waste and chemicals, sloughing layers of dead skin (which can weigh up to a pound!), reducing your sympathetic dominance, and strengthening your immune powers.

Action item. Create your own bathing ritual, once a week.

Step 4: Keep Your Mouth Clean

Brushing and flossing, flossing and brushing. We've had their importance drilled into us since we were kids, but not all of us take care of our teeth and gums the way we should. If you don't yet have a solid ritual, especially with flossing, let this allergy makeover be one more gentle reminder to make one. Inflammation of the gums, gingivitis, and other oral diseases burden your immune system and body and make it that much harder to eliminate allergy symptoms.

In addition to stressing the importance of brushing and flossing, I also want to give you some techniques to keep the whole mouth clean. They will help you remove plaque, bacteria, and chemicals that concentrate in the mouth, so your body can focus its energies elsewhere.

1. FLOSS AND GUM PICK. No surprises here. Flossing, as your dentist has always maintained, is the single most important dental hygiene practice you can do for your teeth and gums. Avoid floss made of plastic and also flavored varieties, which are usually coated with synthetic chemicals.

You'll also want to get a rubber gum pick. It's a wand with a pointed rubber tip at one end, and you can find it with the toothbrushes in any drugstore. While flossing takes care of plaque *between* the teeth, a gum pick is vital for removing anything that gets stuck between the teeth and gums. To use it, simply run the rubber tip along the teeth where they meet the gums, just under the edge of the gums. You'll be moving it in a series of arcs, following the gum line of each tooth. Rather than swallow the debris that is loosened up, rinse your mouth with water, and spit. This largely neglected aspect of dental hygiene will help fight gum disease and inflammation and ultimately reduce oral microbes and microbial toxins that can contribute to your allergy issues.

2. OIL PULLING. Oil pulling is an ancient Ayurvedic practice for daily oral and dental hygiene that involves swishing and "chewing" sesame oil. It is based on the simple principle that oil will collect microorganisms and fat-soluble chemicals (mercury, pesticides, and so on) that collect between our teeth, between teeth and gums, and throughout the oral cavity. It is a painless and powerful technique to help lower your overall toxic burden. For proper oil pulling, you will need one tablespoon of unroasted organic sesame or sunflower oil. For fifteen to twenty minutes, "chew" the oil while swishing it around in your mouth and between your teeth. It will turn into a whitish thick emulsified liquid. This consistency is an indication that the process is complete.

Important: *Afterward, do not swallow the oil! Flush it down the toilet.* The chemicals and heavy metals that have built up in your teeth and gums, as well as the microorganisms in your mouth, have now leached into the oil, so don't swallow it, and don't spit it down the sink. Spit it into tissue without letting it touch your fingers and flush it down the toilet. Rinse your mouth out with warm water, and there is no need to brush your teeth after. It's a simple, cost-effective, all-natural way to keep your mouth clean and refreshed! Try it once or twice a week or even daily.

3. BRUSHING. The best toothbrushes are motorized, with rotary movements designed to loosen and remove food debris, fungi, bacteria, and plaque. Whenever possible, use fluoride-free toothpaste (covered in Day 2). Many companies now offer all-natural toothpastes, which you may find at your local drugstore or supermarket. If not, get them at any health food store or online.

Action item. Buy unroasted sesame or sunflower oil, a gum pick, a motorized rotary-action toothbrush, and all-natural, fluoride-free toothpaste.

Step 5: Move It!

Want one good reason why exercise helps your allergy symptoms? *Sweat.*

That's right, good old-fashioned perspiration is one super allergy fighter. When your body sweats, your pores open and release toxins and other chemicals built up in your system. It's the principle behind saunas, baths, and steam rooms: the more you sweat, the more you detoxify, and less toxic load in your body means less burden on your vital organs and immune system.

When we exercise our large muscles, our metabolism increases and our body temperature rises. Sweating is our natural way to cool off and reduce our core body temperature. Exercise also gives us the added bonus of burning fat for energy, and guess where most toxins, including heavy metals, get stored? In your *fat*! Yes, fat is where our body naturally holds the toxins. It makes sense, considering that fat is not a tissue essential for immediate survival (such as heart or lung tissue). As you exercise, you burn fat. And when you burn fat, toxins are sequestered and you sweat them out. Then it's good-bye mercury, good-bye VOCs, good-bye pesticides; definitely a win–win situation to reduce allergies!

> Fat is where our body naturally holds the toxins.

But getting you to sweat isn't the only reason to exercise. Regular exercise enhances circulation of blood and lymph. These two forms of circulation help you eliminate toxins by moving them from one part of the body to another and preparing them for excretion through the major organs such as the kidneys, liver, and digestive system. With poor circulation, toxins and allergens can get stored in tissues and build up in your body, their harmful effects persisting day after day. Blood flow benefits from the pumping action of the heart, so getting your heart rate up—whether through exercise or by falling in love—will help flush out the chemical buildup.

The lymphatic circulation doesn't directly benefit from the heart's pumping power even though it is a key regulator of the immune system, transporting white blood cells and triggering disease responses. To help your lymphatic circulation, there are at least three things you can do. The first is the use of showers, bathing, and saunas (covered earlier in this chapter) because hot water helps stimulate it. The second is massage, which we'll cover in a bit. And, of course, the third is exercise.

To eliminate toxins, you'll also want to increase the oxygenation to your cells. Along with the dietary changes outlined in Day 1, exercise is your best tool. Increased oxygenation allows your body to facilitate a chemical process (oxidation) that helps break down toxins so that they can react with enzymes and be carried off for elimination. Oxidation "simplifies" toxins so you can sweat them out or excrete them.

And the best reason for exercise? It feels good! Sure, after a few weeks or months of not exercising, it can be a little rough to get going. The joints are creaky, your shoes don't seem as comfortable as they used to, and even a thirty-minute walk can leave you drained. But exercise increases the production of serotonin, a neurotransmitter that makes us happier and leaves us feeling positive about the day ahead. Other than maybe getting a new puppy, I can think of nothing better for our emotional lives than regular exercise. A less reactive emotional system (or, in simpler terms, having more fun) also means a less reactive body, lowering your susceptibility to allergens.

So how do you get back on the wagon after you've fallen off? And how do you stick with the exercise routine you are implementing now? Here are my tips:

1. **FIND SOMETHING YOU LOVE.** Not something you like, feel OK with, or could do for a month, but something you thoroughly *love doing*. My goal here isn't to turn you into a hard-body or a gym rat. If you like the gym and enjoy the focus it gives you, by all means, go! If you enjoy the morning spin class, go for it!

But too many people equate exercise with running on treadmills or hitting the streets in leggings and a sweatband. This kind of workout is not for everyone. But that doesn't mean you can't exercise. What we need to do is think of exercise a bit more broadly, and you will see that there *is* something for you.

Let's say you love gardening but don't have a backyard, because you're renting an apartment. Does that mean you can't use that activity for exercise? No. You can join a community garden in your neighborhood or volunteer with an organization to plant vegetables or help with reforestation efforts. Then, instead of doing what feels like grueling, unsatisfying exercise, you're simply engaging your body in activities you love. And that's good for your mental well-being, too.

You are limited only by your imagination. If you've always wanted to learn to dance, take a salsa class. Learn to surf or go swimming in the ocean. Household projects such as washing all the windows or building furniture in the garage can certainly count as exercise. Jogging with the dog is an easy way to get some exercise while doing something you needed to do anyway. Early morning yoga or Pilates is great, but so is shooting hoops with your kids.

However, the single best form of exercise, which almost everyone can do, is also the most natural one: walking. It's easy and low impact compared to running or competitive sports. It's what we adapted to do when we were hunter-gatherers in prehistoric times. Our bodies really are meant to be lean, mean walking machines because our species developed on the road, walking dozens of miles each week. You might say we have a genetic predisposition to walk! Use a pedometer to see if you can reach a total of ten thousand steps per day. I use one that automatically downloads my daily stats: the number of steps, flights of stairs, distance in miles, and calories burned. Walking for even thirty minutes five times a week will boost your circulation, help you sweat out toxins, increase oxygen to your cells, and help reduce your allergies. It's also good for losing weight (remember, fat is where many toxins and allergens are stored) and strengthening your cardiovascular system.

To prevent depletion and energy loss, it's best to exercise in the morning, when your cortisol levels are at their peak.

But no matter what you decide to do, the key is to engage your body in doing an activity you love. And what's true for exercise is true for life: find something you love, and you will want to do it more often. What once was a struggle is now a joy.

2. DO MANY DIFFERENT ACTIVITIES. I don't want you to think you have to stick to a single activity for the rest of your life. I mean, not all of us were meant to salsa in five-inch heels seven days a week!

In fact, I think it's often best to have a few different activities or classes that you do each week to mix things up. Take a long nature walk on Sunday, do a household project after work Tuesday, and go to the salsa class every Thursday night. Mix in a walk or two, or just spend time running around with the kids, and your week of exercise is complete. Doesn't sound too bad, does it?

3. BE ACCEPTING WHEN YOU DON'T EXERCISE—THEN GET BACK TO IT. Everything's going good. You've hit the trails, downward-dogged, nailed some three-point shots, and ridden the biggest waves this side of Oahu. Great.

But then something happens. Maybe you get sick; maybe there's an issue in the family. Work gets a little extra stressful or you have to go visit the in-laws. By the time things come back to normal, you're not as motivated to get back on the basketball court or the yoga mat. The allure of point breaks no longer calls you, and even the verdant woods seem a little gloomy. Slowly but surely, your exercise routine falls off. You get a little more sluggish, and before you know it, the only exercise you're getting each week is from flipping through the channels with the remote.

We've all been there. And it's OK. Let me repeat, it is totally OK! Yes, you can beat yourself up for being a lazybones if you like, but that only makes getting back into exercise more of a struggle.

It might work for a little while, but in the long run, fighting yourself isn't going to work.

The other option is to accept that you haven't been exercising and get back to your routine as soon as you can. If you find yourself in this situation, here's my best advice: Go easy on yourself. Accept the fact that you haven't exercised in five days, five weeks, or five months. Whatever happened in the past is gone, and it's time to refocus on the present. To start exercising again after a hiatus, I suggest taking some time to think about your most important goals in life again: overcoming your allergies, feeling happy and healthy, fulfilling your dreams and aspirations, whatever they may be. Consider the role that exercising and feeling good about your physical well-being plays in all those goals. Instead of battling to get back to the gym, feel what it would be like to have that same energy, passion, and vibrancy you did when you were exercising and moving. Exercise will help your body heal and give you the energy to focus on what's most important in life.

It might be slow going. You might take only one walk a week for a bit. But as you reconnect with your body and become engaged in things you love, you will begin to have the desire to do more and more. Exercise makes you happier, which makes you want to exercise more. When times get tough, your serotonin will be there to encourage you!

Action item. Exercise for a half hour today. Have fun doing it! Exercise at least three times a week.

Step 6: Get Some Sun

Now that you're exercising, why not add a little sunlight, too? Being out in the sun greatly contributes to our wellness and allergy resistance. If you don't think sunlight contributes to your happiness, you haven't spent a winter in Seattle or Stockholm! Like exercise, sunlight also helps increase serotonin levels, so you feel happier and your nervous system is less reactive.

Sunlight is also one of our main sources of vitamin D because the body uses ultraviolet rays to synthesize it in our skin. Vitamin D promotes healthy immune modulation, and a more balanced immune system means an easier job of handling allergies. With eight- to ten-hour workdays during dark winters in northern latitudes, getting your daily intake of sun can be a challenge.

Here are a few suggestions to maximize your exposure to that celestial light: first make sure your arms and legs are exposed, and then enjoy your morning herbal tea on your terrace before work. Meet your best friend for lunch at an outdoor café, and exercise outdoors whenever possible. A day on the treadmill might be good for your circulation, but a walk along the shore will get the blood flowing *and* help your vitamin D production.

If you live in an especially cloudy (Portland), rainy (Seattle), or snowy (Minneapolis) city, getting enough sunlight daily will be important to prevent a condition called seasonal affective disorder (SAD). Those of us weathering the long, dark winter months in the Northern Hemisphere are especially prone to it. The farther north you are, the worse it can be, especially around New Year's, when daylight lasts only a few hours. Symptoms of SAD may include fatigue, depression, cravings for sugar and carbohydrates, and mental fog.

Winter Blues in Sunny California?

When I started my chiropractic practice in 1989, my first office was in Westwood, Los Angeles, not far from my alma mater, UCLA. I was very excited to start in this location because it was a few blocks away from my gym. I moved into the new office during the summer, and within five months I was not my usual cheery, energized self. I was tired and emotionally depressed for no reason, wanted to sleep during the day, and didn't want to engage socially. I was isolating myself and didn't want to exercise. I took blood tests, and doctors wanted me to take an antidepressant for my symptoms.

That winter holiday, instead of our typical vacation to the mountains for snowboarding, we headed for the warm ocean and balmy breezes of Hawaii. I felt as if that vacation saved my life! Within three days of being in the sun, my depression lifted. It was as if a veil had been lifted off of my head and I was alive again! My energy came right back, and I was back to my old upbeat self.

When I got back from vacation, I researched the correlations between sunlight, serotonin levels, and mood. I was amazed at how prevalent seasonal affective disorder was, even down in sunny southern California! Being my curious detective self, I started to study how many hours of sun I got during my workdays. Five days a week, I worked from seven in the morning to seven at night, in an office with no windows. Worse, I ate my lunch inside, so for five days a week I never got to see or be in the sun (or even *see* it!). No wonder everything went downhill soon after I started my practice. What did I do to get more natural light? I changed my work schedule immediately— started to run around my neighborhood in the early morning and ate my lunch at the local park. I also started using a full-spectrum light visor that emitted full-spectrum light frequency into my eyes to help regulate my serotonin and melatonin production. I have not experienced SAD since, and to this day, twenty-four years later, I still use a full-spectrum lamp from October through March. I have put many of my patients on the same regimen, and many of them swear by it, as I do.

If that sounds like par for your wintertime mood, buy a full-spectrum, or natural, light box or a light visor and use it daily to increase your light exposure. It just may be your cure for the winter blues.

Action item. Spend at least a half hour in the sun today. Buy a light box if you need one.

Step 7: Get a Massage

One type of therapy that can help alleviate allergy symptoms and asthma is getting regular massages to the neck, shoulder, and upper back muscles, particularly around the shoulder blades. Massage can reduce lymph congestion, clear out antigens, lower inflammation, and boost immunity. The less the body is blocked and inflamed, the more attention it can direct toward allergy relief. A better immune system will also help eliminate allergens and toxins more quickly. Massage can also improve your circulation, lower your cortisol levels, and increase your serotonin levels just as exercise does, all while you lie flat on your stomach listening to Enya.

If possible, go to a trained professional at least once a month. Not all forms of massage are the same. You may prefer Thai, Swedish, Shiatsu, or something else. Be sure to do some research beforehand and see what suits you best. When your body starts acting up with symptoms, don't be afraid to start a self-massage routine at home. It doesn't have to be overly complicated, either—just check out a few websites and follow their recommendations. Work your shoulders, feet, back, head, neck, and hands. And if you are suffering from premenstrual syndrome (PMS) or abdominal cramps, you can massage your abdomen, too.

One type of massage I highly recommend for allergy symptoms helps with lymphatic drainage. As your body processes allergens, bacteria, viruses, and toxins, these can build up in your lymphatic channels and nodes, increasing the viscosity of the lymphatic fluid. When you're sick, lymph nodes get swollen from all the bacteria or viruses you're trying to deal with. And if you have allergies, your lymphatic system can be overworked because of all the compounds your body is recognizing as hostile and trying so hard to excrete. You might not have swollen lymph nodes, but the fluid itself can be clogged or blocked with allergens, inhibiting proper circulation and movement. Lymphatic massage will help you drain your lymphatic system and get it back on track.

On each side of your throat, you will find a large muscle running down toward your collarbone. You can find this muscle easily—just turn your head to the right, and the muscle will bulge out on the left side of your neck. This muscle is called the sternocleidomastoid muscle. Put your fingers on each side of this muscle and run them downward, as if you were pushing something down a clogged tube. Don't push too hard, and do this for ten or fifteen minutes. Then we want to activate the lymphatic system just under the collarbone. You can warm it up by gently beating on this area "gorilla style" with your knuckles. Next, rub this area in circles with your fingers and do the same pushing motion that you did with your neck. This massage will help move those toxins out of the lymphatic system to where your body can excrete them properly. You can find even more massage styles for whole-body lymphatic drainage online. You can also find a video on my website called the "Body Balancing Technique," where I show you how to activate your body through tapping various areas in a sequential manner. By tapping these special points, you will activate your lymphatic system, energy points, and physicality. See the resources section, page 263.

Action item. Get a massage. Incorporate weekly massages for lymphatic drainage.

Step 8: Breathe!

The Vedic traditions of India have known about the vital importance and power of breathing for thousands of years. The breath truly is the midway point between body and mind, between the inner and outer world. It is an automatic process of our body that we can control to ensure calm, focus, and peace. More and more people have come to understand the importance of breath through yoga, meditation, or simple mindfulness practices. Also, medical science confirms this ancient understanding: that by breathing deeply and slowly, we can improve our emotional and physical health. So how do we make the most of our breath? Read on!

    1. QUIT SMOKING. If you are smoking cigarettes, you need to stop as soon as possible. I know this isn't easy. I also know that there isn't one surefire solution that works for everyone. Alas, it isn't within the scope of this book to offer thorough guidelines on how to kick a nicotine addiction. But I will recommend that you check out other books and engage your family and friends, counselors, and other supportive members of your community. Let them know you want to quit as part of your allergy health, and get them involved in your process. Simply put, allergy relief cannot really begin if you are still smoking. No amount of organic vegetables and purified water can counteract the onslaught of toxic chemicals inhaled with each cigarette or the damage done by the smoke itself. Such direct exposure to toxic chemicals is overwhelming for someone already trying to cope with pollen, food, or mold allergies. Smoke can lead to allergic reactions such as eye irritation and stuffy nose. It can also damage the nasal passages and bronchial tissues, which are your first line of defense against inhalant allergens.

    The good news is, I have helped many patients quit smoking by weaning them off slowly. If you've tried other methods and they haven't worked, do try this one.

Here is how we do it:

On the first day of the weaning down program, I ask the patient to put however many cigarettes he or she smokes on average a day into a small paper bag. Ten cigarettes a day, a full pack or two, it doesn't matter. That will be their daily allowance of cigarettes per day from now on. If they decide to smoke less, fantastic, but the amount in the bag is all they get for the day. Every four days I ask them to take two cigarettes out of the bag, decreasing their daily allowance. This slow weaning-down process usually does not cause any overt detoxing symptoms such as irritability, fatigue, food cravings or constipation that can come with cold-turkey quitting. It helps most smokers get down to two to four cigarettes a day easily so that completely quitting becomes a breeze. Although it may take a longer amount of time to completely quit, patients are so happy and proud that they have been able to reduce the amount of cigarettes they smoke, feeling healthier and more energized along the way.

If you do decide to quit smoking, I honor you for it. I know that it can be a very tough process. I also know that it is the single most beneficial thing you can do for your allergies and your overall health.

2. BREATHE THROUGH YOUR NOSE. Why should you breathe through your nose? For starters, your nose is a much better filter and purifier than your mouth. Nasal hairs catch pollen and soot. Sticky mucus captures dander and dust. Your nose then warms the air before it enters your lungs and bloodstream, making the oxygen easier to use for life's vital functions. The nose is evolutionarily crafted to fend off allergens, so cherish it and use it!

Many times, breathing through the mouth comes about because of nasal congestion resulting from food allergies. The three main culprits—dairy, gluten, and sugar—are exactly the foods we hoped to eliminate on Day 1. So if your nose feels congested or you are experiencing sniffles or postnasal drip, redouble your efforts to cut out that yogurt, toast, soda, and pastry today. I also recommend spending a bit of time, perhaps each morning, to do a breathing check-in. If you have a regular meditation or yoga practice, you're probably doing something similar already.

Simply spend three to five minutes breathing slowly and deeply *from the diaphragm* and through the nose. Become aware of your breathing and slow it down, allowing your system to calm itself. Pay attention to the inward and outward movement of the diaphragm. Put your hand on your abdomen. It should be expanding and bulging out when you breathe in using your diaphragm muscle. When you exhale, the abdomen should naturally flatten. Chest breathing, on the other hand, gets less air in your system and can actually result in higher anxiety and stress. It's what people do too much of when they hyperventilate. By becoming aware of your breathing patterns, you can return more readily to deep, restful breathing, helping you stay centered and calm. For more information on diaphragmatic breathing, check out the resources section, page 263.

Action item. Quit smoking. Take deep breaths from your diaphragm. Breathe through your nose.

I can say that Day 6 may be the most difficult chapter to fulfill, not because of how many steps it involves but because each step requires a great deal of courage and personal time. Getting exercising and moving again can be difficult and painful at first. If you are a smoker, quitting a lifelong habit takes a great deal of willpower. Bathing once a week may be close to impossible for you; a footbath may be all you can afford in your busy schedule.

Looking for all-natural cosmetics takes effort and energy, and you may need to try several brands to find the right shade, the right quality. You may need to go to the natural pharmacy several times to find the exact shampoo and conditioner that works for you.

If there is resistance to start something new, remember to put each activity into your daily schedule. Give it a specific time and place in your life and it will get easier for you to follow through and master it. Having a routine makes everything easier. Having a routine, paradoxically, gives you freedom.

It takes courage and strength to transform yourself to a healthier new you. You are almost there, and I know you can do it— Day 7 will turbo-charge you to another level of energy and spirit to finally complete your allergy makeover!

CLEAN UP YOUR
STRESS

This is it, the last day of your 7-Day Allergy Makeover. Strange though it may seem, you've made it! After today, you will have all the knowledge and skills you need to live allergy free.

I'm sure the going hasn't always been easy. Maybe you put off getting the shower purifier or recycling all your nonstick pans. You may even have read the first six days and stuck to them vigilantly but are only now reading this final chapter a year later. However you got here, honor your journey and know that your determination and desire for a new life have brought you this far. Although, in one way, today is the last day of your journey, in another way, it's just the beginning. Yes, after today, you will have all the knowledge you need, but I'm sure you will spend the next weeks and months fine-tuning what you've learned and putting more and more of it into daily practice. You might start with a regular gym routine only to realize later that you really want to spend more time on the dance floor or hiking. You might try a particular kind of allergen-free pots and pans only to realize it isn't the best for your family's needs. Fine-tuning your routine will help you adapt to what you've learned in this book, so that it becomes more comfortable and more natural over time. Instead of having to feel these changes as foreign to your life, you want to work to make them a seamless part of the texture of your everyday existence.

Today is really just a beginning in yet another way too. Quite frankly, it can be very difficult to implement all these changes in just a week's time. In fact, I'd be more surprised if you *did* follow this program to the letter than if you had a few hiccups along the way. But what's most important is that each day, you're sticking to the *spirit* of the journey. If you still haven't cut out wheat products entirely, see if you can reduce your intake this week. If you're still using plastic food storage containers, go to the store and buy some glass ones. Take stock of where you are on the journey to allergy-free health, and take note of what you still need to implement from all that you have learned.

At some point, you're likely to find yourself slipping back into old habits. Maybe just for a day, maybe two. Maybe for weeks at a time. Remember that this is OK! Accept the rough patches that come with making deep changes to years and years of old habits. Note where you're having difficulties and just work your way back toward an allergy-free lifestyle. During tough times, you may want to return to the book and reread a key chapter. Check over your notes and underlined sections. Reread the section headings and remind yourself of *all* the changes you hope to integrate into your life. And most important, keep the big picture in sight. Think what it would mean for you to live allergy free: a new energy, a new vitality, and a new opportunity to live the life you want. Finally, rely on your friends and family. If you're about to give up, share your frustrations—as well as your successes—with the people you trust. Be sure to have strong allies in your corner who truly want to see you healed and happy again. If you're not feeling drastic changes right away, don't worry. You've spent years building up your toxic load and entering into a state of sympathetic dominance. Change can be painful, and meaningful change takes time. However, most people who implement all the techniques detailed in this book should begin to feel better within *weeks*, not months or years. No matter what you're going through, it's important to try to reach a place of calm, acceptance, and tranquility.

Life is stressful enough when you don't have allergies playing havoc with your physical and emotional well-being. With allergies, it can feel a hundred times more stressful. This final day covers how to deal with the emotional and mental stress that life throws your way. Workplace stress, family stress, relationship stress. Although I'm not going to give you tips for a better relationship with your spouse or how to get that nagging coworker to relocate to the Outer Hebrides, I am going to give you ways to help your body relax and cope with such external stressors. This chapter helps you develop the centeredness, focus, and tranquility to deal more smoothly and effectively with the challenges we all face.

SYMPATHETIC DOMINANCE: THE EMOTIONAL LINK TO ALLERGIES

Today, I want you to take time to focus on yourself as a *total person*: body, mind, emotions, and spirit. The first six days of your allergy makeover looked at how allergic reactions stress your body's immune, respiratory, and digestive systems and how they can be detrimental to your skin, liver, lungs, nerves, and more. We saw how these physical triggers build up over time, making your body more and more vulnerable to all sorts of allergens, toxins, chemicals, and microbes. In the end, your allergies put your body in a perpetual fight-or-flight state known as *sympathetic dominance*. In such a state, all sorts of triggers, from the people around you to your work environment, to the challenges you face each day, can become harder to handle emotionally. And the result is even more stress and more susceptibility to allergens. You're left with a psychosomatic feedback loop between allergies, physical stress, emotional stress, and more allergies.

Hungarian endocrinologist Hans Selye was the first researcher to understand stress in modern terms. He believed that stress in an urban environment is a prolongation of this fight-or-flight mode. However, instead of experiencing it for a few seconds while we flee that hungry lion, we have come to experience stress for days and days at a time. Instead of a ten-second encounter with a predator, we now face a month-long threat of unpaid bills, credit card debt, or high-demand work environments. When these demands start to add up, the body feels as if it were in physical danger. You could say we have two-million-year-old brains trying to face twenty-first-century problems.

In the prehistoric past, a stress response helped us run faster or summon the energy to grab the nearest rock and hurl it with all our force. Now the adrenaline rush continues on a low level day after day, even when the reason for our stress isn't around. We go back to the same stressful office, feel the burden of our mortgage, and worry about our children's performance in school. Over time, the adrenaline rush that stress produces starts to wear you and your adrenal glands down. At a primal level, it's as if your body were constantly trying to fight off lions on the primeval savannah. Who wouldn't be worn down by that? And in today's world, unlike on the African savannah, the lions of stress never disappear. Every day presents a new challenge, a new issue. And as your body wears down from adrenal overload, you become less able to deal with allergens. *Emotional stress produces allergic sensitivity.*

To deal with this feedback loop, the first step is to deal with the allergens. Mold, pollen, dander, plastics, heavy metals—you name it. And that's exactly what the first six days of the allergy makeover have done. But we can also reverse the feedback loop of sympathetic dominance from another angle. What if we work to heal your emotional stress as a way of making your body less reactive to allergens in the first place? What if we focus on your breath, your feeling of connectedness with nature, and your ability to be present as ways to bring back your body's inner calm and centeredness? As you begin to undo sympathetic dominance, allergens that would have bothered you before lose their power over you. Situations that once made you feel defeated, powerless, or inadequate become mere *challenges*, to face from a place of self-assurance and confidence.

> Emotional stress produces allergic sensitivity.

But let's be clear: This chapter is not a self-help guide. Self-help books tend to focus on changing your thought patterns or emotional reactions using a set of psychological principles. And although some of my clients have found such books helpful, the changes the books produce can sometimes be short-lived. Once the principles of the book are forgotten or no longer implemented, old ways of thinking return. Old emotional patterns recur, and this is especially true for people with allergies. Why? Because sometimes the changes these books recommend simply don't go deep enough. To make profound and lasting life changes, it's not enough merely to *think* differently—you must *embed* life changes in the body. Your body itself must begin to feel, act, and respond to the world in a new way. For example, you may try to become more accepting of negative thought patterns, but what if these thought patterns come from a deeper disharmony in your physical system? What if your body is, in fact, at war with itself? How can you become a more generous, accepting person at an emotional level if every day is a struggle at the most basic physical level?

To create a new emotional life, you must virtually create a new body.

That said, I certainly do value the work that is done by counselors, mentors, psychologists, and spiritual advisers throughout the world. The

> To create a new emotional life, you must virtually create a new body.

path of lifelong self-awareness and personal growth, is certainly one of the worthiest that you can travel. And the time, understanding, and energy that such teachers and coaches devote to the people who seek out their help simply can't be replicated here. What this chapter *can* do, though, is help you reduce the stress you feel, by working on the breath, using movement, and reconnecting with activities you love. The importance of the mind–body connection cannot be overstated. By making joyous, invigorating activities a part of your physical routine, you come to expect joy and vitality *emotionally* as well. As you take time for yourself and get in touch with the physical world around you, your emotions respond. The more carefully you attend to the physical sensations you are feeling, and the more care and compassion you lavish on your body, the more care and compassion will fill your emotional life as well.

Before we jump into the techniques for dealing with emotional stress, let's take a look at some of the stressors that are very much a part of our everyday lives.

Workplace Stress

Americans are some of the hardest-working people in the world. It's just a fact. But this isn't entirely a good thing. Our insatiable work ethic, our equating of life with work, our willingness to put in sixty or even *eighty* hours at the office is turning out to be a mixed blessing. Want to know what the number one stressor of most Americans is? According to a survey by Mental Health America, "nearly half of Americans (48 percent) are stressed by finances," and another 32 percent are stressed by "workplace issues," such as problems with coworkers, or unemployment.[1]

When work becomes the main focus of life, everything else falls by the wayside. Our need to move and exercise, our longing for solitude and reflection, our desire to connect with others and be part of a larger community—all can fall prey to a culture that values hard work above all else. As a culture, we tend to be very results oriented. Instead of focusing on how much joy we get from what we are doing or how we are improving the world, we tend to look at whether a job will help us move to a better neighborhood, upgrade our car, or pave the way for a better retirement. The end result is that *living* gets lost in the process.

And while work can certainly be rewarding, many of us feel that we are simply trapped in a job that isn't fulfilling. *Forbes* magazine ran a story about a survey in which Right Management found out that only 19 percent of respondents were completely satisfied with their jobs.[2] Two-thirds of respondents were actually *dissatisfied*. A similar study by Mercer shows that, at any given time, 32 percent of us are actually looking for different work.[3] Too many of us feel stuck in something our hearts aren't invested in. We may just be going through the motions so we can pay the mortgage and buy groceries. Worse still, our talents and skills go underutilized and underappreciated. We are reluctant to talk with coworkers or superiors with whom we don't see eye to eye, which only adds to our stress. We accept overwork and under-payment and lose a sense of balance between life and work. Adrenal exhaustion and a state of sympathetic dominance have now become the norm. Allergies often follow—a worn-down body has a more difficult time dealing with allergens, and stress can reduce the concentration of friendly gut bacteria needed for optimal digestive health and to keep unhealthy microbes at bay. And this process can drag on for years until we scarcely recognize what is going on.

I hope that you can begin to get a sense of where your life may be out of balance, and what you can do to fix it. Do you have commitments that you may be able to let go of so you can spend more time focusing on yourself? Is your job a part of your emotional burden? Are you lacking a real connection with your friends, family, and community? Can you enlist those around you to help out with more of the chores and household responsibilities so you can get back in touch with your body and your feelings? At the end of the day, focusing on yourself is not selfish. Restoring your body to its inherent vibrancy will make you more generous with your time and more open with your feelings. The more your body can relax, the more *you* can relax, and the more patience, energy, and under-standing you will have to offer others.

Health-Related Stress

Besides work, the main stressors that most Americans face are those related to their health. I'm sure this comes as no surprise. You wouldn't be reading this book if you didn't know more than most people just how grueling living with health issues can be. Allergies are tough enough to handle, but unfortunately, they of-ten lead to a whole host of other ailments. Being in a mode of sympathetic dominance leads to a weaker immune system, and so infections and colds have an easier time targeting you. It's rare to find someone who has allergies but is otherwise in perfect health. The systems that allergies affect are so closely related to your overall health that, where there are allergies, diseases are almost bound to follow. By breaking the cycle of allergies, you give your body a better chance to fend off colds or flu when they come your way.

And if you are lucky enough *not* to have serious health issues other than your allergies, you may have family members struggling with cancer, heart disease, arthritis, or a host of other ailments. It's stressful to watch our grandparents, parents, and other loved ones suffer. It's even harder still when we don't feel they are getting proper care. Medical bills and the debts incurred from hospital care are the number one reason for bankruptcy in America. Every day, too many of us are walking a tightrope, hoping not to get seriously injured or sick. I have been working in the healthcare field for twenty-four years, and I am utterly convinced that the best form of medicine is *preventive* medicine. This allergy makeover won't cure all diseases. But every guideline in this book is not just good for your allergies; it's also good for your long-term health. By following them, you and your family will be healthier and better able to deal with disease than ever before.

Relaxation or More Stress?

We all know how important it is to spend time by ourselves and relax. But many of the activities we use to relax—watching television, drinking alcohol, browsing the Internet—may actually be at cross purposes with deep and lasting stress reduction. In fact, some of these activities may actually contribute to long-term stress rather than alleviate it. Alcohol is a perfect example. While it may relax us in the short term, it's also a depressant and a diuretic, is harmful to the brain, can contribute to insomnia, is hard on the liver, and has a high sugar content. Moreover, it adds to your toxic load and, therefore, harms your ability to deal with allergies. Short-term relaxation comes at a cost to long-term allergy health. But what about television, incessant Web browsing, or playing video games? Ask whether you engage in these activities from a conscious decision or simply because you need a distraction from the *real* underlying stress. I'm not saying you shouldn't play your favorite video game, check Facebook, or catch up on the last season of *Game of Thrones*. But it's important to understand what is actually prompting you to do it. You may be doing something because stress has put you on mental autopilot, or you may be doing it because you are living in the present moment and *choose* to do it. There's a huge difference between doing something as a distraction and doing something rejuvenating that you truly love.

NATURAL STRESS RELIEF

So how do we learn to live without being so badly shaken and worn down by the stresses of work and poor health? How do we break this cycle of sympathetic dominance that wears our bodies down? How do we become centered and tranquil at the deepest level? We can't all quit our jobs and become surf bums. From Day 6, you already know the healing effects that sunlight, massage, bathing, and exercise can have on your mood. But I'm going to give you some more techniques to help your body relax. These are some of the best ways to work on the psychosomatic connection to emotional health. And that means better allergy health.

Step 1: Wake Up Slowly and Stretch

Have you ever watched a dog wake up? Or a cat? If not, you should sometime. What you'll see is nature's way of greeting the new day. Millions of years of evolution have refined this morning ritual, and it's worth watching just so you can see how far we humans have strayed from it. Our hypothetical dog—let's call him Rex—will open his eyes slowly, blinking a few times. The world hasn't yet fully entered his consciousness. Blood is slowly returning to his higher cognitive faculties, reminding him where his food bowl is and pricking his ears with the sounds of a squirrel scampering across the roof. The first thing you'll see Rex do is stretch out his legs as far as possible. Then he'll probably go back to just lying there. After all, what's the rush? For the next few seconds, he probably won't make any sudden movements—won't seem to be doing much of anything. After a bit, he might stretch out his legs some more. Give him a minute or two, and Rex will work his way to his feet and do a bit of yoga. That downward dog position is called that for a reason! Dogs (and cats, too) love to wake up their bodies by giving their limbs and back a moment to come back to life. Stretching and taking everything slow and easy is the best way to do that. Finally, Rex licks his fur for a few moments to tidy up. Ready for another day of chasing cats, scaring mail carriers, catching tennis balls, and just relaxing, Rex is about as happy as a dog can be.

Now let's compare Rex to his typically American human, named Tom. At 7:00 a.m., Tom hears the alarm and presses the snooze button, trying to fend off reality. Already, even in this half-awake state, he starts thinking about the stresses of life. Five minutes pass, and he hits the snooze button again. After doing this four or five times, Tom realizes that he's stretched it to the last possible minute if he doesn't want to be late for work. He snaps out of bed, throwing the covers on the floor, and staggers toward the coffeepot. Even before eating, he downs a cup or two and heads to the shower. Instead of bathing carefully, he has barely time for a military shower. On a good day, he grabs something to eat on the way to work. But on days like this, forget it—no time for breakfast. He rushes into the office, almost late for a meeting. By the time 10:00 rolls around, he's headed to the office pastry pile for the morning sugar-and-carbohydrate overload. An hour or two later, he feels himself crashing from the sugar and caffeine, so he tries to offset the crash with another cup of coffee, which lasts another hour or two.

Let's see what we can do to reverse this trend. First, even if it means waking up earlier, *take time to wake up.* No more snooze button, and no more jumping to your feet at the last possible second. Instead, lie in bed for a few extra minutes and allow yourself to exist in that dreamy half-awake state. Allow the body to warm up slowly, like a car on a cold morning. Wait for the blood to get flowing and the brain to blink on. Even your computer takes a few moments to boot up—you should, too.

Second, connect with your body. Does it feel relaxed and calm or can you feel your stress in certain parts of your body? Are you congested when you wake up? Are your eyes itchy and watery, or moist and healthy? Do you have postnasal drip or irritation in the back of your throat? In other words, before hitting the shower, do what I call a body scan, where you check to see how your allergies have progressed and whether you're feeling any new or unexpected aches and pains. Chart this progression over the next few days as you make it part of your everyday regime.

Third, take time to stretch every morning. Most stretching you can even do in the comfort of your own bed. Use your intuition and listen to what your body needs. Stretch an arm or a leg, or simply tighten and relax your muscles. You can also do the lymphatic drainage massage from Day 6. This need not be a full-on gym-style stretching routine. It's just a way to get the blood flowing and your body feeling alive and awake. From the body scan, determine which muscles may need extra attention. If you want to maximize the benefit of this routine, I suggest you review stretching or yoga postures online and try them out for yourself. Fifteen minutes of stretching will help get the joints, muscles, and nervous system ready for the day. Also, by breathing slowly while you stretch, you increase blood flow and will feel calmer. If it works for Rex, it can work for you, too.

Finally, see if you can take a bowel movement in the morning to rid your body of bloating and waste buildup. You will feel lighter as you set about your day, and you won't be as stressed. If you have difficulty taking a bowel movement in the morning, drink hot water with lemon, herbal tea, or decaffeinated coffee to help stimulate your digestive tract. To improve regularity, up your intake of fiber, water, and anything with probiotics (healthy bacteria). Fermented foods such as kimchi, coconut yogurt, miso soup, and sauerkraut are great options. You can also take probiotic supplements in powder or capsule form.

Action item. Wake up slowly, connect with your body and its sensations, and stretch lightly.

Step 2: Create a Routine

You've probably heard about circadian rhythms or an internal biological clock. But what do these terms really mean? Your body has a natural rhythm, with times for waking, sleep, eating, and eliminating. It expects to do certain things at certain times because hormones appropriate to each kind of activity get released at the appropriate times. It wouldn't make sense for your body to release the hormones that scream "Energy rush!" at 11:00 at night, and so it doesn't. By that time, your body expects to be calming down or relaxing (if not asleep already). Everybody differs somewhat, within a spectrum. The morning is for excretion, eating, and activity. In the evening, you are not set up to handle as much food as during midday. At nighttime, of course, your body expects relaxation, not a third round of martinis at the local bar.

To honor your body's rhythms, the best thing you can do is create a routine. When you do something at a time the body doesn't expect, the body gets a bit of a shock. "I wasn't expecting a bacon cheeseburger at two a.m.!" The harmony between physical activity and the endocrine system is thrown out of whack. But if you do the same thing at the same time day after day, the nervous system will adapt and expect certain shocks (such as exercise) at certain times, and other activities (such as eating) at other times. The body then becomes better able to handle these stresses because it is properly prepared. While you can set up your own routine, the ideal strategy is to follow the body's innate rhythms—the ones that came programmed in your genes. We are truly creatures of habit, right down to our DNA.

For these reasons, it's vital to pay attention to your eating habits. Too many of us work through lunchtime, skip breakfast, or eat dinner in the wee hours of the night. On certain days, this may be unavoidable, but if your eating routine is not having a routine, it's time to reconsider. I'm going to suggest that you eat every three to four hours (three times a day, plus a snack) to keep your blood sugar level in balance. Skipping meals (or eating too much sugar) will ultimately lower your blood glucose levels, causing adrenaline and cortisol to kick in. That means your body is trying to "rev you up" with hormones because you haven't eaten. In our primal environment, this made sense. But in our modern world, when most of us aren't in danger of imminent starvation, we want to prevent this up-and-down cycling of adrenaline and cortisol. Too much adrenaline wears down the system and, yes, leads to more sympathetic dominance. By eating regularly and keeping balanced blood sugar levels, you can reduce your anxiety, irritability, and emotional stress. You stay calmer and have natural, vibrant energy without the need for caffeine or sugar to pick you up.

One final tip: in your tablet or smartphone, schedule your day to help you stick to this regular routine. Plan to eat breakfast, and plan to leave the office for lunch. Give yourself time to exercise and time to wind down at night. Make sure your routine includes your meals, work hours, exercise, time with the family, sleep, and, most important, *time to yourself.* To get a more detailed example of how making a schedule and following your natural biorhythms can work for you, read my articles on my website, the7dayallergymakeover.com.

Structure Creates Freedom

Forty-two-year-old Carol complained of both digestive and respiratory allergies. The mother of four young children, she was always tired and exhausted. She felt that she did not have much time for herself at all and was often tearful and overwhelmed. Every minute of her life went to taking care of her children and husband. Before she became a mother, she was a full-time lawyer, and now she often secretly wishes she was working again because the job of mothering was so much more difficult and stressful. Carol said she didn't have time to exercise or to spend with her husband. She often skipped eating meals, and a couple of times a week she even skipped taking a shower! Having four young children, all under the age of ten, was a formidable responsibility, even with a full-time nanny and a housekeeper. Frazzled and declining from allergies and fatigue, she felt that her body was now starting to break down.

Looking at Carol's current lifestyle, I knew I could give her only a few simple tasks to help her allergies and energy level. I did ask her to remove only two foods from her diet: dairy and gluten products. I felt that giving her any more instructions would only burden her by adding more stress to her already fragile state, rather than relieving her. The most profound way to help Carol was to get her on a healthy daily schedule that was practical and reasonable.

We scheduled mornings as the best time to get her walk and yoga classes in. The nanny would take care of her toddler for two hours Monday, Wednesday, and Friday. We wrote it out on her Daily Schedule form so she could actually *see* her routine. The form is available to download at the7day allergymakeover.com/resources. We scheduled her weekdays and weekends completely, from the moment she woke up until bedtime. We scheduled into her day only all her basic priorities: her showers, meals, walks, carpools, and even her daily water and supplement intake. I asked her not to add into her schedule *anything* extra, such as movies with friends or volunteering for charity events, so that we could restore her body and spirit and build a reserve of energy and vitality.

Once I showed her that preparation is essential and that we could deliberately create her day with purpose and clarity, she felt that she could follow it because of its simplicity. For the following two weeks, Carol followed her daily schedule to the letter.

At her next appointment, Carol said that her energy level had doubled, roughly from a 3 to a 6, on a scale from 1 to 10. Eating smaller meals and chewing her food slowly, combined with eliminating the worst of the fermentable carbohydrate

foods (dairy and gluten), helped considerably with her digestion, easing the bloating and flattening her stomach down to
her prepregnancy size. Her nasal congestion and sinus pressure
went away, and she began to feel more energetic and even
experienced a renewed sex drive. Above all, having a schedule
gave her a new sense of focus and purpose because she could
do what she loved and make time for all her familial obligations. With a schedule, Carol felt she had a *purpose* to her life
as a mother and wife and, most important, a purpose to being
herself. She was doing everything she loved to do and wanted
to do, and with the structure, she actually felt more freedom.
The thought of going back to work as a lawyer was the fur-
thest thing from her mind, because she was filling her life with
purpose by deliberately creating her day.

So many changes in such a short period of time, just by
scheduling her day! Now, with some structure in her schedule
and biorhythms, her body felt relief and built up a reserve of
energy, and she was ready to tackle a complete 7-Day Allergy
Makeover. She was motivated to make more changes, to have
the healthy life she deserved.

Action item. Create a daily schedule and write down your routine including meals, meetings, exercise, and relaxation times.
Structure creates freedom.

Step 3: Create a Daily Reminder for Tasks

Has your mind ever run on an endless loop? You're at work and you
get a thought pattern like this: "I have to pay the bills. How much
money do I have? When do the kids get done with soccer today?
Do we have anything to eat in the fridge? Oh, boy, the living room

is a mess. I have to work on getting it to look better," and so on. You go back to work for a little bit and notice that you're stressed out. Why? Because a thought pattern starts up: "I really need to pay the bills. How much money do I have?" You know the rest. This cycle of thinking without taking action can result in procrastination, forgetting tasks, and, of course, stress. The truth is, our brains weren't designed to handle multiple complex tasks all at once. It's very easy to get overwhelmed when your life involves dealing with children, work, shopping, paying bills, and a hundred other responsibilities.

Here's the secret truth: Our brains are great at planning and executing small, discrete tasks such as "I need to go get postage stamps." But think how much harder it is for our brain to process more abstract endeavors such as "I really need to upgrade my living room." Planning the first task is easy: Get in the car, drive to the store or post office, and pay for stamps. But when we are faced with something as complex as "upgrade my living room," the task seems overwhelming. That's because so many factors and considerations can potentially go into upgrading a living room, the brain doesn't know how to deal with that degree of complexity. You push the thought away only to find, ten minutes later, that it's back. So what can you do? Short of telling your family you can take care of only one task per day (wouldn't that be nice?), the best plan is to *segment all your larger tasks into smaller ones and write them down.* Nothing stops the mental loop as quickly as writing down specific tasks that your brain can actually handle.

The benefit of this method, besides reducing mental stress, is that you can easily plug these activities into a calendar so you're more likely to do them. "Improve the living room" might sound like a weekend project. But "look on the Internet for upholsterers" can be a ten- or fifteen-minute process. It also means you can start your project right away. At work, we use our calendars to remind us of meetings, deadlines, and other tasks. Why not do the same for your household projects, your responsibilities, *and* your free time? Segmenting activities and planning externalizes these thoughts so that our minds become available for other issues. That walk in nature isn't fun if you're worrying about the need to check your bank account. When you write it down, your mind lets go of that concern, knowing that it can always turn to your planner to remind it of everything you need to take care of. That's why I think it's so important not just to plan things for work but also to plan times for relaxation, eating, and work breaks. One of the easiest ways to get caught in stressful habits is *not to allow* yourself to take the time you need to enjoy the things you love, to meditate, to enjoy the sunshine, and to be present with your family and with yourself.

Action item. Segmenting activities will free your mind. Single tasking clarifies your intention!

Step 4: Be in the Present and Do What You Love

There are few times in life when we are intensely in the moment. Falling in love is certainly one of those. It can also happen the first time you drive a car or during a great run or while watching the sunset. But being in the present isn't just for exquisite or singular experiences, nor is it the exclusive preserve of enlightened beings and spiritual masters. If you already have a meditation practice, much of this will be familiar. If you haven't yet tried meditation or mindfulness practices and have even an ounce of curiosity, I encourage you to try. They are great for slowing down your thought patterns (including those endless loops) so that you can witness them with more detachment. When that happens, you become less attached to the thoughts that create stress and anxiety. You see them for what they are: thoughts that give you information about your current emotional state but will soon pass—thoughts that can be acted on or left to fade away. Either way, *you* are the one deciding how to react to them. Your thoughts are no longer controlling your every action. Instead of being in that runaway train known as your habitual thought patterns, you are the one in the driver's seat, using thoughts as helpful road maps.

The most commonly practiced form of mindfulness is a breathing meditation. To do this, simply become aware of your breath. You may concentrate on the rising and falling of your diaphragm, the air entering and going in and out of your nose or your full body breathing. Feel your breath as it enters and leaves your body. Naturally, thoughts will come up that distract you. Simply witness them with a playful curiosity and acknowledge them. Then, without judging your thoughts, just return to witnessing your breath. You *will* have your attention wander away. That's not a problem. It's just what the mind does. Just notice that your mind has wandered, and accept it, returning always to the breath. Even a three-to-five minute mindfulness check-in can work wonders if you do it a few times a day. After that, you may wish to extend your sessions gradually to fifteen or twenty minutes.

But being in the moment can be as simple as paying attention to life as it is happening. Maybe you're eating a juicy apple. Maybe your boss just dumped a pile of papers on your desk. OK! Both are great times to practice mindfulness. With more focus, you *can* be more fully present in both those moments. Slow down as you eat and become aware of the apple. What are the textures of the apple, the sensations of sour and sweet that it gives you? Is it rough or smooth? How do you feel about this new workload? Agitated? Frustrated? Overwhelmed? Is it a new opportunity or challenge? Where do you feel the stress? In your neck, back, or shoulders? Does your whole body feel tense? Wherever you are, being present, witnessing and accepting the emotions and thoughts that come your way is the best way to live fully in the moment. When you become distracted or begin identifying with your thoughts, simply bring yourself back to the present moment and the sensations and feelings in your body. Mindfulness is simply a practice of noticing and paying attention, which you can do anywhere. Practicing mindfulness can certainly help your feelings of centeredness, calm, and poise. For a more extensive explanation, I highly recommend checking out some of the many books and websites that discuss its benefits.

For most of us, however, the *easiest* way to become more present in the moment is to do what we love doing. Doing what we love puts us in contact with life and *nothing else.* For that moment, there are no bills to pay, no broken car, no fridge full of wilting vegetables. There's almost no better way to experience calmness and vitality than by experiencing what you deeply love. That's why scheduling it into your life (see step 2) is absolutely vital to your allergy makeover. Too often, we skip doing what we love, because life gets in the way. That habit ends today. Every week, I want you to make time to practice what you love, as much as you possibly can. Some weeks, it may be only an hour. On weeks with fewer obligations, it could even be a whole weekend or more. But the days without the activities you love are over, because your allergy health demands that you enjoy your life.

........................◯........................

Your allergy health demands that you enjoy your life.

........................◯........................

Finding such timeless experiences will be different for everyone. For some people, hiking in nature allows them to appreciate the wonderful biodiversity of our planet. Someone else might experience rapturous joy swimming in the ocean or simply playing with their dog. For you, it might be playing the clarinet, gardening, sculpting, or something else. And it doesn't have to be something grand. The key is *being in your body in the present moment.*

Our best experiences come from these meditative moments. Meditative moments are the opposite of the fight-or-flight responses. They are the moments when we feel no pressure, no rush, and no sense of worry. They are the way to overturn the rule of sympathetic dominance.

Action item. Engage only in activities that you love to do and that bring joy into your life. Connect to your breath and recognize what your body is feeling at the moment. Practice mindfulness to help you feel centered and calm.

Step 5: Try Earthing

Have you ever taken a barefoot walk on the sand or a stroll on the grass and felt a warm energy in your feet? Have you ever felt more grounded when some part of your body senses the earthly elements: raindrops on your face, your feet in the cool river, your connection with the warmth and hardness of a boulder as you watch the sunset, the heavy scent of sage while hiking in a canyon? If your answer is yes, then you already know something of the power of earthing. Earthing is, quite simply, the process of getting your body back in touch with the earth and its inherent energy. Our ancestors spent every moment of their lives barefoot and connected to the earth and nature. Our bodies adapted to receiving electrical energy from the earth, and it remains beneficial to our wellbeing and sense of belonging and place. Our modern style of walking with plastic shoes and synthetic socks, fully clothed, wearing sunglasses and sunscreen, can leave us feeling disconnected and anxious.

If you're skeptical, just try this exercise. Go somewhere free of thorns, glass, or other hazards—say, a beach, expanse of lawn, or maybe a botanical garden—and take a barefoot walk. Check how you feel beforehand and how you feel afterward. Notice whether you feel any sort of warm or tingling sensation in your feet. The walk can be as short as fifteen minutes (but while you're at it, why not get your exercise in for the day, too, and make it thirty or forty-five minutes?) At the end of the walk, notice whether you feel any release of tension, discomfort, or pain. Do you feel more alive and connected with the world around you?

I'm a big fan of earthing—so much so that I even carry two smooth river rocks with me when I travel to medical conferences. I rest and massage my feet on the rocks while listening to presentations or stand on them in the hotel room after being indoors all day. Of course, with outdoor venues, you don't even need the stones—just a patch of grass will do. Earthing immediately connects me to a bit of natural earth once again. I live in the Santa Monica mountains, so when I hike, rather than just strolling in the woods, I "nature bathe." The wild natural setting engages all my primal senses, and I instinctively connect to my deep, intuitive self. I listen to the movement of the trees and grass around me and smell and feel the energy of the mountain. The fresh negative ions in the air hug me gently. Try earthing. I'm betting you won't be disappointed.

Action item. Get grounded by walking barefoot on grass or the beach.

Step 6: Make Time for Yourself

Finally, I want you to make a commitment to spend a half hour by yourself every day. This can be a mental, emotional, and physical check-in to see how you feel during your 7-Day Allergy Makeover. It will help you be in the present and make you aware of what bodily and emotional stresses you may be experiencing.

This process isn't easy. You're going to be feeling new things, thinking new ideas, and dreaming new dreams. You'll need some time for self-reflection, for self-understanding. Use this time however you please, so long as you are alone and in the moment. You can sit in your favorite chair and feel the state of your body. How are your allergies today, and how were they yesterday? What did you do to help them, and what can you do tomorrow to help them more?

This may be your time for prayer, meditation, or introspection. It can be a time for journaling or writing about the transformative process you've embarked on. You could lie in bed with a book about natural health, or simply practice deep breathing. Whatever you choose, this is your time *for you*. In the end, you have only one body and one life. By making time for yourself, you are honoring that body and that life as you see best. This is your time to listen to your heart, see your dreams in all their fantastic Technicolor, and ponder where you want to go. To learn more about meditation and mindfulness, including how to practice it, check out the article on my website.

Action item. Create time for self-reflection and journal about your dreams, goals and transformations.

FINAL NOTE

I wrote this book for two reasons. First, I have been fortunate to be able to help thousands of people in southern California transform their lives through my 7-Day Allergy Makeover program, which wakes up the body's inner healing abilities to restore it from inside out. People who thought they were doomed to a life of rashes, coughing, sneezing, fatigue, bloating, indigestion, headaches, and worse made a decision to heal themselves naturally and permanently—to break free from their allergies so they can enjoy a brilliant, bold, and exceptional life.

By following the 7-Day Allergy Makeover, you too have been affected by your body's powerful innate ability to heal and free yourself from allergies. I can only imagine the hardship you've gone through and what brought you to this point. I want to honor those difficult years of suffering and, now, all the efforts you've made during the course of reading and implementing the steps in this book. It's not always easy to choose to change your life. But you've made that decision, and for that, you have my deep admiration.

Second, I believe that only by having a healthy body can we truly be at peace mentally, emotionally, and with the world and environment around us. Only by having a healthy body can we be our best selves. We can begin to think about how we can truly help our families, our communities, and our ecosystems. In other words, as you leave behind your allergies, I sincerely believe that you can begin to live with even more generosity, openness, and freedom.

And from there, who knows what can happen?

ACKNOWLEDGMENTS

Writing this book was so much easier than finding the words to express my undying gratitude to the people who supported and stood by me during this amazing journey as a mother, wife, doctor, student, colleague, and, now, author.

As I think of how to express my thanks to my dear son, Cody, feelings of a mother's love well up inside me. To help him in his struggle with allergies, I learned the value of healthier, all-natural solutions, which have now benefited hundreds of my patients.

Thank you, Cody, for all that you went through. I appreciate your patience and understanding of the many weekends I spent away at conferences and seminars to learn more about allergies and natural medicine. You are the love of my life. Thank you so much!

To George, my wonderful, loving husband and life partner, I am eternally grateful that we met twenty years ago while riding our Harleys on Sunset Boulevard! Thank you so much for being my greatest cheerleader and champion. No matter what I wanted to do, learn, and participate in, you always gave me the space to experience my life to its fullest.

I want to express my endless love and gratitude to my mother, Sarah Chun. Thank you, Mom, for your kindness and generosity. I deeply respect your supreme wisdom and strength. You are truly the queen of Korean mothers. You nourished our spirits with your life stories and with your out-of-this-world delicious Korean meals. Dad, I am forever grateful to you for teaching me two of my strengths: flexibility and perseverance. I don't think I would have finished this book without these qualities, and I know your spirit is right there encouraging me to move forward. You are always in my heart.

To my siblings, Lisa, Chuck, and Maggie, thank you so much for all your love and support. I am *so* lucky to have you in my life. And to Cory and Craig, my stepsons, I am so thankful that Cody has you as his big bros. We love you. Big hugs and kisses to my tribe: Rose Pinard, Fariba Kavian, Lavinia Errico, Heather Hayward, Dawn Alane Kelmenson, and Kimberly Truman—my dearest girlfriends whom I love and adore. I am so grateful to have you in my life. Thank you all for teaching me how to be a woman, mother, wife, sister, and friend.

I am in deep gratitude for the friendship and support I receive from my mastermind groups: Center Ring and Integrative Practice Wellness members. A special shout-out of love and appreciation to my Rockstar Docs group: Hyla Cass, Joan Rosenberg, Grace Suh, and Nalini Chilkov, as well as to Marcelle Pick, JJ Virgin, Alan Christianson, Mikell Suzanne Parsons, Anna Cabeca, Sara Gottfried, Jonny Bowden, Steven Masley, Habib Wicks, Jennifer Landa, Todd LePine, and Charles Sophy—you all continue to inspire me with your vision, passion, and enthusiasm.

Thank you so much, Frank, for all that you do for our Wellness for Life Center—you keep the practice running smoothly and efficiently, with sincere enthusiasm and peerless customer service skills, especially with children. We all love you!

I am so proud of my protégé, Dr. Karen Liu—you have been a superstar with my patients, your acupuncture skills are amazing, and I am excited to witness your growth as a practitioner.

I want to give my warmest thanks my two mentors: JJ Virgin and Brendon Burchard. JJ, thank you so much for believing in me and seeing something that I didn't know I had: a desire to share my work with a bigger audience. Your tenacity and strength are infectious. You are truly a feminine warrior! Brendon, thank you for being the most influential person in my life this past year, both in personal growth and in business practices. You have inspired me to be the best person I can be, so I can share my message with authenticity, passion, and service. The first time I met you, at Experts Academy 2012, I stood up and asked you in front of eight hundred people if I should publish my ebook online or take a big chance and submit a book proposal to the traditional publishing houses. And without hesitation, you told me to go for it. Well, Brendon, I did it!

My deep and warmest thanks to Zen, Michael, and John for being so readily available and helping me with my editing, research, and book proposal. You guys are brilliant people, and I couldn't have done it without you.

To my publisher, Perigee, and amazing editor in chief, Marian Lizzi, thank you so much for believing in me and my desire to share my voice on allergy health. Words cannot describe how much our collaboration means to me. Thank you from the bottom of my heart for giving me this phenomenal opportunity. And a special shout-out to your incredible team of editors and publicists, as well as the marketing department, graphic designers, and assistants—your commitment is greatly appreciated!

I will never forget my literary agent, Coleen O'Shea, for her support and insight during the whole process of creating this book. Thank you so much for everything. I know you will always have my back! And special thanks to my dear friend and colleague Jonny Bowden, for introducing us.

I am deeply indebted to the American Academy of Environmental Medicine and its teachers, including Dr. Doris Rapp, Dr. Sherry Rogers, and Dr. William Rea. I am also grateful for all my incredible teachers and mentors of natural, homeopathic, Oriental, functional, and integrative medicine. Over twenty-four years of postgraduate work, I have taken hundreds of classes and seminars, so I can't mention every teacher, but I do want to acknowledge Dr. Devi Nambudripad. I thank you every day for opening my eyes to the power of healing. All of you have sparked my quest to dig deeper and learn the root causes of allergies. Without your insight, wisdom, and generosity, I would not be the natural allergist I am today.

I am forever grateful to all of my patients—thank you for believing in the process of true healing, the all-natural way. I honor you for your dedication to feeling better and restoring optimal health and vitality. To the parents of my pediatric patients—I honor you for your perseverance in finding the right but sometimes difficult journey for your children's health. Often going the unconventional medical path can be met with resistance and without social support, but know that I am here for you, to facilitate your growth as an allergy-free family! I want to give special thanks to my out-of-the-country and out-of-town patients and to the hundreds of families from San Diego, for traveling long hours to see me. I am endlessly dedicated to your wellness and health goals.

And finally, I would like to thank the readers for having the courage to open up my book and start a comprehensive approach to healthy, allergy-free living. Start slowly, but dig deep. Being your own allergy detective is most rewarding and empowering.

Thank you for giving me this opportunity to serve you and your loved ones. My desire is to help you feel better, the all-natural way, so you can be brilliant and bold and live an exceptional, healthy life full of energy and vitality.

Be well.

Very truly yours,
Dr. Susanne Bennett

APPENDICES

ALLERGY SYMPTOMS CHECKLIST

DIGESTIVE TRACT

❏	Nausea and vomiting		❏	Belching or passing gas	
❏	Loose or pasty stool		❏	Stomach pain or cramps	
❏	Diarrhea		❏	Heartburn or acid reflux	
❏	Constipation		❏	Blood and/or mucus in stools	
❏	Bloated feeling				
				TOTAL	

JOINTS AND MUSCLES

❏	Pains or aches in joints		❏	Swollen, tender joints	
❏	Arthritis		❏	Growing pain in legs	
❏	Stiffness or limitation of movement		❏	Gout	
❏	Pain or aches in muscles		❏	Fibromyalgia	
❏	Feeling of weakness or tiredness				
				TOTAL	

HEAD

❏	Headaches		❏	Facial flushing	
❏	Faintness		❏	Facial numbness	
❏	Dizziness		❏	History of head trauma	
❏	Insomnia, sleep disorder				
				TOTAL	

SKIN

❏	Acne		❏	Hair loss	
❏	Itching		❏	Flushing or hot flashes	
❏	Hives, rash, dry skin				
				TOTAL	

EYES

❏	Watery or itchy eyes		❏	Red, swollen, or sticky eyelids	
❏	Bloodshot eyes		❏	Bags or dark circles under eyes	
				TOTAL	

EARS

❏	Itchy ears		❏	Reddening of ears
❏	Earaches, ear infections		❏	Excess ear wax
❏	Ringing in ears		❏	Ear tubes
❏	Hearing loss		❏	Drainage from ears
				TOTAL

NOSE

❏	Stuffy nose		❏	Hay fever
❏	Postnasal drip		❏	Sneezing
❏	Chronically red, inflamed nose		❏	Excessive mucus formation
❏	Sinus problems			
				TOTAL

MOUTH AND THROAT

❏	Chronic coughing		❏	Swollen or discolored tongue, lips
❏	Frequent clearing		❏	Canker sores
❏	Swollen tongue, teeth marks on side of tongue		❏	Itching on roof of mouth
❏	Sore throat, hoarseness, loss of voice		❏	Gagging
				TOTAL

WEIGHT AND APPETITE

❏	Binge eating or drinking		❏	Water retention
❏	Craving certain foods		❏	Lack of appetite
❏	Hungry in the middle of the night		❏	Feeling of fullness
❏	Compulsive eating		❏	Excessive weight
				TOTAL

ENERGY AND ACTIVITY

❏	Apathy, lethargy		❏	Restless leg syndrome
❏	Attention deficit		❏	Poor physical coordination
❏	Fatigue		❏	Low libido
❏	Insomnia		❏	Stuttering, stammering
❏	Hyperactivity, restlessness		❏	Slurred speech
				TOTAL

EMOTIONS

❏	Mood swings		❏	Unwarranted fear
❏	Anger, irritability, aggressiveness		❏	Feelings of overwhelm
❏	Anxiety, nervousness		❏	Frustrated, cries often
❏	Argumentative		❏	Depression
				TOTAL

MIND

❏	Poor memory		❏	Difficulty completing projects
❏	Confusion		❏	Difficulty with mathematics
❏	Easily distracted		❏	Difficulty making decisions
❏	Learning disabilities		❏	Poor/short attention span
❏	Underachiever in school		❏	History of brain trauma
				TOTAL

LUNGS

❏	Chest congestion		❏	Persistent cough
❏	Asthma bronchitis		❏	Wheezing
❏	Shortness of breath		❏	Air hunger
❏	Difficulty breathing		❏	Sleep apnea
				TOTAL

HEART

❏	Irregular or skipped heartbeat		❏	Heart murmur
❏	Rapid or pounding heartbeat		❏	Valve disease
❏	Chest pain			
				TOTAL

OTHER

❏	Frequent illness		❏	Antibiotics as a child
❏	Vaccine reactions		❏	Eat fish/seafood more than twice a week
❏	Mercury fillings			
				TOTAL
				GRAND TOTAL

BODY COMPOSITION TRACKING SHEET

Name:	Weight (lb.):	Height (in.):	BMI: weight ÷ height × 703
Main issue(s):		Pulse rate (bpm):	Blood pressure (mm Hg):

Measurements:		
	Before	After
1. Biceps *(upper forearm)*		
2. Chest *(level with nipple line)*		
3. Waist *(level with belly button)*		
4. Hips *(level with pubic bones)*		
5. Thigh *(3 inches below pubic bones)*		

Photos: include photos of before and after	
Before	Before
After	After

ALLERGY-FREE FOOD SHOPPING LIST

It is best to buy organic fruits, vegetables, grains, legumes, nuts/ seeds, oils, etc. Look for animal protein that is organic, grass-fed, free-range, cage-free, and free of antibiotics and dyes. Eat fish or seafood only once a week, due to the excess mercury, nuclear waste, and other toxins in our oceans today. My food list is only a recommendation; do not eat any foods listed if you are intolerant or allergic to them.

Proteins

FROM LAND
Lean Poultry
- ❑ Chicken
- ❑ Duck
- ❑ Game hen
- ❑ Turkey

Eggs
- ❑ Chicken
- ❑ Duck
- ❑ Goose
- ❑ Quail

Lean Beef
- ❑ Chuck steak
- ❑ Extra-lean hamburger
- ❑ Flank steak
- ❑ Lean Veal
- ❑ London broil
- ❑ Top sirloin steak
- ❑ Any other lean cut

Lean Pork
- ❑ Pork loins
- ❑ Pork chops
- ❑ Any other lean cut

Game Meat
- ❑ Bison (buffalo)
- ❑ Elk
- ❑ Goat
- ❑ Goose

- ❑ Muscovy duck
- ❑ Ostrich
- ❑ Pheasant
- ❑ Quail
- ❑ Rabbit

- ❑ Squab
- ❑ Venison
- ❑ Wild boar
- ❑ Wild turkey

FROM SEA
Fish (Wild Caught)
- ❑ Anchovies
- ❑ Branzini (Mediterranean sea bass)
- ❑ Cod (scrod)
- ❑ Flatfish
- ❑ Haddock
- ❑ Herring
- ❑ Mackerel

- ❑ Monkfish
- ❑ Mullet
- ❑ Red snapper
- ❑ Rockfish
- ❑ Sablefish
- ❑ Salmon
- ❑ Sardines
- ❑ Striped bass

Shellfish
- ❑ Abalone
- ❑ Crab
- ❑ Lobster

- ❑ Scallops
- ❑ Shrimp

Other
- ❑ Octopus
- ❑ Sea cucumber

- ❑ Skate
- ❑ Squid

VEGETABLES
- ❑ Artichoke
- ❑ Arugula
- ❑ Asparagus
- ❑ Beet greens
- ❑ Beets
- ❑ Bell peppers
- ❑ Broccoli
- ❑ Brussels sprouts
- ❑ Cabbage
- ❑ Carrot

- ❑ Cauliflower
- ❑ Celery
- ❑ Chives
- ❑ Collards
- ❑ Cucumber
- ❑ Dandelion
- ❑ Eggplant
- ❑ Endive
- ❑ Frisee
- ❑ Garlic

- ❑ Ginger
- ❑ Green onions
- ❑ Kale
- ❑ Kohlrabi
- ❑ Lettuce
- ❑ Mustard greens
- ❑ Onions
- ❑ Parsley
- ❑ Parsnip
- ❑ Peppers
- ❑ Pumpkin
- ❑ Radish

- ❑ Rutabaga
- ❑ Seaweed/sea vegetables
- ❑ Snow peas
- ❑ Spinach
- ❑ Squash
- ❑ Swiss chard
- ❑ Tomatillos
- ❑ Tomato
- ❑ Turnip greens
- ❑ Turnips
- ❑ Watercress
- ❑ Zucchini

FRUITS

- ❑ Apples
- ❑ Apricots
- ❑ Avocado
- ❑ Banana
- ❑ Blackberries (frozen)
- ❑ Boysenberries (frozen)
- ❑ Blueberries (frozen)
- ❑ Cantaloupe
- ❑ Carambola (starfruit)
- ❑ Cherries
- ❑ Cherimoya
- ❑ Cranberries
- ❑ Dragon fruit
- ❑ Gooseberries (frozen)
- ❑ Grapefruit
- ❑ Guava
- ❑ Honeydew
- ❑ Jujube

- ❑ Kiwi
- ❑ Lemon
- ❑ Lime
- ❑ Lychee
- ❑ Mango
- ❑ Nectarine
- ❑ Orange
- ❑ Papaya
- ❑ Passion fruit
- ❑ Pears
- ❑ Pineapple
- ❑ Peaches
- ❑ Persimmon
- ❑ Plums
- ❑ Pomegranate
- ❑ Raspberries (frozen)
- ❑ Rhubarb

HERBS

- ❑ Basil
- ❑ Chili
- ❑ Coriander/cilantro

- ❑ Lemongrass
- ❑ Marjoram
- ❑ Mint

❑ Oregano
❑ Parsley

❑ Rosemary
❑ Thyme

OILS/BUTTERS

❑ Avocado oil
❑ Coconut oil/butter
❑ Flaxseed oil/butter
❑ Grapeseed oil
❑ Macadamia nut oil
❑ Olive oil

❑ Perilla oil
❑ Sesame oil
❑ Walnut oil
❑ Hemp seed butter
❑ Chia seed butter

NUTS AND SEEDS

❑ Almonds
❑ Brazil nuts
❑ Chestnuts
❑ Chia seeds
❑ Flaxseed
❑ Hazelnuts
❑ Hemp

❑ Macadamia nuts
❑ Pecans
❑ Pine nuts
❑ Pumpkin seeds
❑ Sesame seeds
❑ Sunflower seeds
❑ Walnuts

LEGUMES

❑ All beans
❑ Black-eyed peas
❑ Chickpeas
❑ Lentils
❑ Miso

❑ Peas
❑ Snow peas
❑ Soybeans
❑ Sugar snap peas

ANCIENT GRAINS

❑ Amaranth
❑ Quinoa

❑ Teff

OTHER HEALTHY GRAINS

❑ Brown rice
❑ Buckwheat (not a true grain, but prepared like a grain)
❑ Millet

❑ Gluten-free oats
❑ Organic corn
❑ Wild rice

BEVERAGES

- ❏ Bottled carbonated spring water
- ❏ Noncaffeinated herbal tea
- ❏ Purified, reverse osmosis filtered water

Most of the foods listed fall in the low-glycemic index category.

GUT RESTORE FOOD CHECKLIST

Eat These Foods Low in Fermentable Sugars

PROTEINS
- ❑ All game meats
- ❑ Beef
- ❑ Chicken
- ❑ Eggs
- ❑ Fish/seafood (once a week)
- ❑ Pork
- ❑ Turkey

FRUITS
- ❑ Avocado (limit ¼)
- ❑ Banana (small)
- ❑ Blueberries
- ❑ Boysenberries
- ❑ Cantaloupe
- ❑ Carambola (starfruit)
- ❑ Cranberries
- ❑ Coconut
- ❑ Dragon fruit
- ❑ Durian
- ❑ Grapes
- ❑ Grapefruit (limit ¼ cup)
- ❑ Honeydew
- ❑ Kiwi
- ❑ Lemon
- ❑ Lime
- ❑ Mandarin
- ❑ Melon
- ❑ Orange
- ❑ Papaya
- ❑ Passion fruit
- ❑ Pineapple
- ❑ Raspberries
- ❑ Rhubarb
- ❑ Star anise
- ❑ Strawberries
- ❑ Tangelo

VEGETABLES
- ❑ Alfalfa
- ❑ Alfalfa sprouts
- ❑ Arugula
- ❑ Bamboo shoots
- ❑ Bean sprouts
- ❑ Beets (limit 4 slices)
- ❑ Bok choy
- ❑ Broccoli (limit ½ cup)
- ❑ Brussels sprouts (limit ½ cup)
- ❑ Butternut squash (limit < ¼ cup)
- ❑ Carrot
- ❑ Celeriac
- ❑ Celery
- ❑ Chives
- ❑ Cucumber

- ❑ Eggplant
- ❑ Endive
- ❑ Ginger
- ❑ Green beans
- ❑ Kale
- ❑ Lettuce
- ❑ Olives
- ❑ Parsnip
- ❑ Peas (limit < ¼ cup)
- ❑ Potato
- ❑ Pumpkin
- ❑ Radish
- ❑ Red bell pepper

- ❑ Rutabaga
- ❑ Scallions
- ❑ Spinach
- ❑ Summer squash
- ❑ Sweet potato (limit ½ cup)
- ❑ Swiss chard
- ❑ Taro
- ❑ Tomato
- ❑ Turnips
- ❑ Water chestnut
- ❑ Yam
- ❑ Zucchini

FRESH HERBS

- ❑ Basil
- ❑ Chili
- ❑ Coriander/cilantro
- ❑ Ginger
- ❑ Lemongrass
- ❑ Marjoram

- ❑ Mint
- ❑ Oregano
- ❑ Parsley
- ❑ Rosemary
- ❑ Thyme

NUTS/SEEDS (LIMIT HANDFUL)

- ❑ Almonds
- ❑ Chia seeds
- ❑ Flaxseed
- ❑ Macadamia nuts
- ❑ Pecans

- ❑ Pine nuts
- ❑ Pumpkin seeds
- ❑ Sesame seeds
- ❑ Sunflower seeds
- ❑ Walnuts

GLUTEN-FREE GRAINS

- ❑ Arrowroot
- ❑ Brown rice
- ❑ Gluten-free bread or cereal products
- ❑ Gluten-free oats
- ❑ Millet

- ❑ Polenta (corn)
- ❑ Psyllium
- ❑ Quinoa
- ❑ Sorghum
- ❑ Tapioca

MILK ALTERNATIVES
- ❑ Almond milk
- ❑ Coconut milk
- ❑ Gluten-free oat milk
- ❑ Hemp milk
- ❑ Rice milk

SWEETENERS
- ❑ Erythritol (small amounts)
- ❑ Stevia

ALL HEALTHY OILS/BUTTERS
- ❑ Avocado oil
- ❑ Coconut oil/butter
- ❑ Flaxseed oil/butter
- ❑ Ghee
- ❑ Grapeseed oil
- ❑ Macadamia nut oil
- ❑ Olive oil
- ❑ Sesame oil
- ❑ Walnut oil
- ❑ Hemp seed butter
- ❑ Chia seed butter

Avoid These Foods High in Fermentable Sugars

FRUITS
- ❑ Apples
- ❑ Apricots
- ❑ Avocado (> ¼)
- ❑ Blackberries
- ❑ Canned fruit in natural juice
- ❑ Cherries
- ❑ Concentrated fruit sources
- ❑ Dried fruit
- ❑ Fruit juice
- ❑ Longon
- ❑ Lychee
- ❑ Mango
- ❑ Nectarine
- ❑ Peaches
- ❑ Pear/Asian pear
- ❑ Persimmon
- ❑ Plums
- ❑ Prunes
- ❑ Watermelon

VEGETABLES
- ❑ Artichoke
- ❑ Asparagus
- ❑ Beetroot
- ❑ Broccoli (> ½ cup)
- ❑ Brussels sprouts (> ½ cup)
- ❑ Button mushrooms
- ❑ Cabbage
- ❑ Cauliflower
- ❑ Chicory
- ❑ Fennel
- ❑ Garlic
- ❑ Green bell pepper

- ❑ Leek
- ❑ Mushroom
- ❑ Okra
- ❑ Onions

- ❑ Shallots
- ❑ Snow peas
- ❑ Spring onions
- ❑ Sweet corn

LEGUMES

- ❑ Baked beans
- ❑ Chickpeas
- ❑ Kidney beans

- ❑ Lentils
- ❑ Soybeans (tofu, tempeh)

GLUTEN GRAINS

- ❑ Barley
- ❑ Couscous
- ❑ Kamut
- ❑ Spelt

- ❑ Triticale
- ❑ Rye
- ❑ Wheat

MISCELLANEOUS

- ❑ Alcohol/beer/wine
- ❑ Chicory
- ❑ Dandelion

- ❑ Inulin
- ❑ Pistachio

ALL MILK PRODUCTS

- ❑ Buffalo milk
- ❑ Cow milk
- ❑ Goat milk
- ❑ Sheep milk
- ❑ Cottage cheese
- ❑ Cream

- ❑ Custard
- ❑ Ice cream
- ❑ Mascarpone
- ❑ Ricotta
- ❑ Yogurt

SWEETENERS

- ❑ Agave
- ❑ Fructose
- ❑ High-fructose corn syrup
- ❑ Isomalt

- ❑ Maltitol
- ❑ Mannitol
- ❑ Sorbitol
- ❑ Xylitol

KEY TERMS

adrenal exhaustion A state of fatigue and potential sleep disruption produced by stress and excessive adrenaline release over time.

allergen Any food, chemical, or foreign substance that causes an allergic reaction.

allergy Any bodily reaction to a nutrient, food, inhalant, chemical, or foreign substance that produces a cellular dysfunction and disturbs the normal physiology of the cell, gland, organ, or system.

anaphylaxis Intense and potentially lethal allergic reaction often characterized by swelling of the throat and lips, hives, and difficulty breathing.

antigen Any foreign substance, including allergens, that the body perceives as a threat.

antihistamine Pharmaceutical used to control the symptoms of allergies. Although they offer temporary relief, such drugs do not address the underlying cause of allergies and may produce unwanted side effects.

bisphenol A (BPA) A potential endocrine disruptor and allergen found in many plastics (usually plastic 7), including in children's toys. Now banned for use in baby bottles.

carcinogen Chemical that can cause cancer through repeated exposure.

casein Potentially allergenic protein found in dairy products.

companion planting Growing of different crops in proximity to assist each other in nutrient uptake, pest control, pollination, or other functions important to crop productivity.

dairy Potentially allergenic food group, including milk, cheese, and yogurt, containing the milk of nonhuman animals. Allergic symptoms often include stomach problems and digestive issues such as constipation, gas, and diarrhea.

dental fluorosis Discoloration of tooth enamel caused by fluoride exposure, often as a result of fluoridated tap water or fluoridated toothpaste.

diatomaceous earth A light silica-containing material, derived chiefly from diatom remains, often crumbled into a powder and used for filtering and natural pest control.

dust A potentially allergenic accumulation of human skin particles, dust mite droppings, pet dander, and fabric lint, often from clothes.

dust mites Tiny arachnids that burrow in pillows, sheets, and other fabrics and consume shed human skin. Some of their proteins, including those in their droppings, can be allergens.

earthing The practice of connecting the human body (often through the feet) to the electrical energy of the earth.

endocrine disruptor A foreign chemical that acts like a hormone in the body and interferes with the normal functioning of the endocrine system. Especially harmful during pregnancy and childhood development. Examples include BPA, PFOA, and phthalates.

endogenous Originating within the body (as, for example, certain chemicals or hormones).

fluoride Chemical compound often added to tap water in the belief that it prevents tooth decay. Potential allergen that, in high enough concentrations, can cause dental and skeletal fluorosis.

gluten Potentially allergenic protein found in many cereal grains such as wheat, barley, and rye and products derived from them, such as bread, pizza dough, bagels, and pastries. Symptoms can include bloating, stomach pain, brain fog, fatigue, low energy, and diarrhea.

hay fever An allergic reaction often characterized by nasal inflammation, itchy, watery eyes, and sneezing. Often caused by allergies to dust mites, pet dander, mold, or pollen.

heavy metals Often toxic, potentially allergenic metals with a high atomic weight. For the purposes of this book, I include silver, nickel, and aluminum, which are often found in cookware, utensils, and other kitchen products.

HEPA filter High-efficiency particulate air filter, capable of eliminating up to 99 percent of airborne allergens.

histamine A compound ($C_5H_9N_3$) that the body releases to deal with allergens and other antigens.

IgE (type I) allergic reaction An acute allergic reaction that produces an immune response and is often characterized by swelling and inflammation, rash, itch, and discomfort.

lactose A sugar in milk that produces allergies in many people.

lymphatic drainage Removal of allergenic and toxic substances from the lymphatic system for elimination. May be accelerated by massage, hot showers, and exercise, among other techniques.

lymphatic system Bodily system that transports white blood cells, helps with immune responses, and traps allergens and other antigens in the lymph nodes.

mindfulness The practice of becoming aware of one's moment-to-moment physical, emotional, and mental sensations and perceptions. Reduces stress and deconstructs sympathetic dominance. Often considered similar to meditation.

molds Fungi that often grow in food or damp, humid areas. Mold is a potential allergen, and symptoms can include exhaustion, rashes, and difficulty in breathing as well as those associated with hay fever.

mycotoxin Compounds produced by fungi that are toxic or harmful to human health.

nitrogen oxides Toxic and allergenic chemical compounds released by combustion processes in many power plants and engines. Among the ingredients, along with VOCs, that produce smog.

nonpoint source of pollution Water pollution that comes from runoff or ambient sources. Motor oil and fertilizers that leach into water sources are examples.

outgas To release trapped gas from a surface over time. Plastics and paints outgas fumes that can be allergenic.

pet dander Skin shed from animals, often pets, which includes potentially allergenic proteins. Often found in dust.

perfluorooctanoic acid (PFOA) Chemical used in making nonstick pans and some packaged foods (such as microwave popcorn), which is potentially carcinogenic. PFOA production has been greatly reduced and is expected to be eliminated altogether because of its adverse health effects.

pollen The male fertilizing agent of plants, often responsible for IgE allergic reactions, including hay fever.

polytetrafluoroethylene (PTFE) Chemical coating used in nonstick pans and pots, which has toxic and allergenic effects.

probiotics Bacteria that benefit healthful bodily functioning. Can be found in many foods (such as kimchi) and some soaps.

proprioception The body's internal perceptions that help it determine location, hand–eye coordination, and balance, among other things.

reverse osmosis A method of cleaning foreign molecules and chemicals from water using pressure on one side of a semipermeable membrane.

sensitivity A state of heightened physical reaction to a molecule or chemical (such as gluten or chlorine) that disrupts cellular function and may trigger an immune response.

sodium lauryl sulfate Potentially allergenic chemical compound used for foaming and cleaning and found in many beauty and hygiene products.

stress A fight-or-flight condition triggered by a stressor and marked by the production of higher levels of adrenaline and cortisol.

stressor Any foreign threat to the body that produces stress. Such threats can include allergens such as gluten or pollen, emotional or interpersonal issues, or fear of bodily harm.

sugar Any sweet simple carbohydrate, such as glucose, fructose, or sucrose, that is a potential allergen and is found in many foods and drinks. Common sources of sugar are candy, soda, alcohol, baked goods, and sweeteners such as honey and agave. Refined grains such as white bread, pasta, and white rice are rapidly converted to sugar in the body. Allergic symptoms can include hyperactivity and anxiety, energy crashes, exhaustion, and joint pain.

sulfur dioxide Toxic compound produced during industrial processes and combustion of many fuels, also used in food preservation. One of the ingredients in acid rain.

sympathetic dominance A physical state defined by a constant fight-or-flight mode, in which the sympathetic nervous system, which is responsible for handling emergencies, controls our daily functioning, resulting in emotional wear, adrenal exhaustion, and difficulty in dealing with allergies.

toxin A chemical or substance that is harmful or potentially lethal to the body.

volatile organic compounds (VOCs) Allergenic, toxic, and potentially carcinogenic organic compounds, such as formaldehyde, methylene chloride, and perchloroethylene, that are found in synthetic products, including some paints, wall coverings, car exhaust, and adhesives and are also used in the dry-cleaning process. When they evaporate, certain VOCs contribute to the formation of smog.

whey The lactose-containing part of milk that remains after curds have been separated. Can be allergenic to anyone sensitive to lactose.

xenobiotics Substances, typically synthetic chemicals, that are foreign to the body or to an ecological system.

RESOURCES

Private Practice

Dr. Susanne Bennett
Wellness for Life Center
1821 Wilshire Boulevard, Suite 300
Santa Monica, CA 90403
Tel: 310-315-1514
Fax: 310-315-1504

Dr. Susanne's Websites

drsusanne.com
purigenex.com
wellnessforliferadio.com
the7dayallergymakeover.com

Dr. Susanne's Social Media

Facebook: facebook.com/drsusannebennettallergyspecialist
Instagram: @drsusanne
LinkedIn: Dr. Susanne Bennett
Pinterest: @drsusanne
Twitter: @drsusanne

Downloads

Go to the7dayallergymakeover.com/resources for:
  Allergy-Free Food Shopping List
  Allergy Symptoms Checklist
  Body Balancing Technique Video
  Body Composition Tracking Sheet
  Daily Schedule Form
  Diaphragmatic Breathing Video
  Gut Restore Food Checklist
  Jumping Rope Video
Fourth National Report on Human Exposure to Environmental
  Chemicals: cdc.gov/exposurereport/pdf/FourthReport_
  UpdatedTables_Mar2013.pdf
Pollen maps: pollen.com

Functional Laboratories

Enterolab: enterolab.com
Genova Diagnostics/Metametrix: gdx.net
  Comprehensive Digestive Stool Analysis: gdx.net/product/10140
  IgG ELISA Food Antibodies: gdx.net/product/10145
  Intestinal Permeability Assessment: gdx.net/product/10122
Glycemic Index: glycemicindex.com
Sanesco: sanescohealth.com

Favorite Books on Allergies and Environmental Medicine

Barnett, Cynthia. *Blue Revolution: Unmaking America's Water Crisis* (Boston: Beacon Press, 2012).

Block, Mary Ann. *No More Ritalin: Treating ADHD Without Drugs* (New York: Kensington, 1996).

Bock, Kenneth, and Cameron Stauth. *Healing the New Childhood Epidemics: Autism, ADHD, Asthma, and Allergies* (New York: Ballantine, 2008).

Colborn, Theo, Dianne Dumanoski, and John Peter Meyers. *Our Stolen Future: Are We Threatening Our Fertility, Intelligence, and Survival?* (New York: Plume, 1997).

Cordain, Loren. *The Paleo Diet Revised: Lose Weight and Get Healthy by Eating the Food You Were Designed to Eat* (Boston: Houghton Mifflin Harcourt, 2010).

Crinnion, Walter. *Clean, Green, and Lean: Get Rid of the Toxins That Make You Fat* (Hoboken, NJ: Wiley, 2010).

David, William. *Wheat Belly: Lose the Wheat, Lost the Weight, and Find Your Path Back to Health* (Emmaus, PA: Rodale, 2011).

Deutsch, Roger, and Rudy Rivera, MD. *Your Hidden Food Allergies Are Making You Fat* (New York: Prima Lifestyles, 2002).

Freinkel, Susan. *Plastic: A Toxic Love Story* (Boston: Houghton Mifflin Harcourt, 2011).

Lewith, George, Julian Kenyon, and David Dowson. *Allergy and Intolerance: A Complete Guide to Environmental Medicine* (London: Merlin Press, 1998).

May, Jeffrey C., and Jonathan M. Samet. *My House Is Killing Me!: The Home Guide for Families with Allergies and Asthma* (Baltimore, MD: John Hopkins University Press, 2001).

McDonald, Libby. *The Toxic Sandbox: The Truth About Environmental Toxins and Our Children's Health* (New York: Perigee, 2007).

Null, Gary, PhD. *No More Allergies: Identifying and Eliminating Allergies and Sensitivity Reactions to Everything in Your Environment* (New York: Villard, 1992).

Perlmutter, David, and Kristin Loberg. *Grain Brain: The Surprising*

Truth about Wheat, Carbs, and Sugar—Your Brain's Silent Killers (New York: Little, Brown, 2013).

Pollan, Michael. *The Botany of Desire: A Plant's-Eye View of the World* (New York: Random House, 2002).

Pollan, Michael. *The Omnivore's Dilemma: A Natural History of Four Meals* (New York: Penguin, 2007).

Price, Weston A., and Price-Pottenger Nutrition Foundation. *Nutrition and Physical Degeneration* (Lemon Grove, CA: Price-Pottenger Nutrition, 2008).

Rapp, Doris J., MD. *Impossible Child* (Practical Allergy Research Foundation, 1989).

Rapp, Doris J., MD. *Our Toxic World* (Environmental Research Foundation, 2003).

Rogers, Sherry A., MD. *Detoxify or Die* (Solvay, NY: Prestige Publishing, 2002).

Schroeder, Henry Alfred, MD, and William J. Rea, MD. *The Poisons Around Us: The Unseen Dangers in Our Air, Water, Cookware and Food, and Their Leading Roles in Sickness* (Chicago: Keats Publishing, 1994).

Skinner, Juniper. *Food Allergies and Me: A Children's Book* (CreateSpace Independent Publishing, 2010).

Steingraber, Sandra. *Living Downstream: An Ecologist's Personal Investigation of Cancer and the Environment* (Cambridge, MA: Da Capo, 2010).

Wilson, Edward O., Rachel Carson, and Linda Lear. *Silent Spring* (Boston: Houghton Mifflin, 2002).

Korean Spas in the United States

Los Angeles, California
Aroma Spa and Sports (Men and Women)
3680 Wilshire Boulevard
Los Angeles, CA 90010
(213) 387-0111
aromaresort.com

Crystal Spa (Men and Women, Co-Ed Room, Open 24 Hours)
3500 W. 6th Street, Suite 321
Los Angeles CA 90020
(213) 487-5600
crystalspala.com

Natura Spa at the Natura Sports Health Club (Men and Women)
3240 Wilshire Boulevard
Los Angeles, CA 90010
(213) 381-2288
natura-spa.com

Olympic Spa for Women
3915 West Olympic Boulevard
Los Angeles, CA 90019
(323) 857-0666
olympicspala.com

Wi Spa (Men and Women, Co-Ed Room, Open 24 Hours)
2700 Wilshire Boulevard
Los Angeles, CA 90010
(213) 487-2700
wispausa.com

San Diego, California
Aqua Day Spa (Men and Women)
4637 Convoy Street, Suite 105
San Diego, CA 92111
(858) 279-8889
aquadayspasandiego.com

Honolulu, Hawaii
Aloha Sauna and Spa (Women Only)
1724 Kalauokalani Way
Honolulu, HI 96814
(808) 941-9494
alohasauna.com

Chicago, Illinois
King Spa & Sauna (Men and Women)
809 Civic Center Drive
Niles, IL 60714
(847) 972-2540
kingspa.com

Palisades Park, New Jersey
King Sauna (Men and Women)
321 Commercial Avenue
Palisades Park, NJ 07650
(201) 947-9955
kingsaunanj.com

New York City Area, New York
Spa Castle (Men and Women)
131-10 11th Avenue
College Point, NY 11356
(718) 939-6300
nyspacastle.com

Dallas, Texas
King Spa & Sauna (Men and Women)
2154 Royal Lane
Dallas, TX 75229
(214) 420-9070
kingspa.com

Centreville, Virginia
Spa World USA (Men and Women)
13830-A10 Braddock Road
Centreville, VA 20121
(703) 815-8959
spaworldusa.com

Seattle, Washington
Olympus Spa (Women Only)
3815 196th Street SW, Suite 160
Lynnwood, WA 98036
(425) 697-3000
and
8615 S. Tacoma Way
Lakewood, WA 98499
(253) 588-3355
olympusspa.com

NOTES

Day 2: Clean Up Your Water

1. Elina Jerschow, Aileen P. McGinn, Gabriele de Vos, Natalia Vernon, Sunit Jariwala, Golda Hudes, and David Rosenstreich. "Dichlorophenol-Containing Pesticides and Allergies: Results from the US National Health and Nutrition Examination Survey 2005–2006." *Annals of Allergy, Asthma & Immunology* 109, no. 6 (2012): 420.
2. Douglas McIntyre, "10 American Cities with the Worst Drinking Water," *Daily Finance*, January 31, 2011. dailyfinance.com/2011/01/31/ten-american-cities-with-worst-drinking-water.
3. Jacqueline D. Savitz, Christopher Campbell, Richard Wiles, and Carolyn Hartmann, "Dishonorable Discharge: Toxic Pollution of America's Waters," Washington, DC, Environmental Working Group, 1996, p. 2. static.ewg.org/reports/1996/Dishonorable-Discharge.pdf.
4. Ibid., p. 1.
5. Ibid.
6. Charles Duhigg, "Clean Water Laws Are Neglected, at a Cost in Suffering," *New York Times*, September 12, 2009. nytimes.com/2009/09/13/us/13water.html?pagewanted=all&_r=0.
7. American Rivers, "Polluted Runoff: Health Effects of Sewage," americanrivers.org/initiatives/pollution/public-health.
8. Crystal Gammon, and OurAmazingPlanet, "Satellites Track Hurricane

Sandy Water Pollution," Scientific American, November 17, 2012. scientificamerican.com/article.cfm?id=hurricane-sandy-water-pollution.

9. U.S. Environmental Protection Agency, "Arsenic in Drinking Water," water .epa.gov/lawsregs/rulesregs/sdwa/arsenic/index.cfm.

10. Fluoride Action Network, "Tooth Decay in F vs. NF Countries," fluoride alert.org/issues/caries/who-data.

11. Eugenio D. Beltrán-Aguilar, Laurie Barker, and Bruce A. Dye, "Prevalence and Severity of Dental Fluorosis in the United States, 1999–2004." NCHS Data Brief No. 53, Hyattsville, MD: National Center for Health Statistics, 2010. cdc.gov/nchs/data/databriefs/db53.htm.

12. UNICEF, "Common Water and Sanitation-Related Diseases," last updated June 17, 2003. unicef.org/wash/index_wes_related.html.

13. Dr. Paul Connett, "50 Reasons to Oppose Fluoridation," *Second Look*, slweb .org/50reasons.html.

14. NoFluoride.com, "Cities Rejecting Fluoridation Since 1990," nofluoride .com/cities_rejecting.cfm.

Day 3: Clean Up Your Air

1. EPA, "Ground Level Ozone: Health Effects," November 2012. epa.gov/glo/ health.html.

2. A. J. Cohen, H. Ross Anderson, Bart Ostro, et al., "The Global Burden of Disease Due to Outdoor Air Pollution," *Journal of Toxicology and Environmental Health* 68, nos. 13–14 (2005): 1301–1307. ncbi.nlm.nih.gov/pubmed/ 16024504.

Day 5: Clean Up Your Kitchen

1. S. Bull and K. Foxall, "PFOS and PFOA—Toxicological Overview," Public Health England, 2009. www.hpa.org.uk/webc/HPAwebFile/HPAweb_C/ 1246260032570.

2. Ibid.

3. Stephen Musson, "Geopedia: Bisphenol A," *National Geographic*, September 18, 2008. ngm.nationalgeographic.com/geopedia/Bisphenol_A.

4. Leonard Sax, "Polyethylene Terephthalate May Yield Endocrine Disruptors," *Environmental Health Perspectives* 118, no. 4 (2010): 445–448.

5. R. Rudel and L. Perovich, "Endocrine Disrupting Chemicals in Indoor and Outdoor Air," Atmospheric Environment 43, no. 1 (2008): 170–181. ncbi .nlm.nih.gov/pmc/articles/PMC2677823.

6. Centers for Disease Control and Prevention and Department of Health and Human Services, "Fourth National Report on Human Exposure to Environmental Chemicals," last updated March 2013, cdc.gov/exposurereport/pdf/ FourthReport_UpdatedTables_Mar2013.pdf.

7. K. Thayer, J. Heindel, J. Bucher, M. Gallo, "Role of Environmental Chemicals in Diabetes and Obesity: A National Toxicology Program Workshop Review," *Environmental Health Perspectives* 120, no. 6 (2012): 779–789.

8. U.S. Environmental Protection Agency, "Nickel Compounds," January 2000. epa.gov/ttnatw01/hlthef/nickel.html.

9. C. Exley, L. M. Charles, L. Barr, et al., "Aluminium in Human Breast Tissue," *Journal of Inorganic Biochemistry* 101, no. 9 (2007): 1344–1346.

10. P. C. Ferreira, A. Piai Kde, A. M. Takayanagui, and S. I. Segura-Muñoz, "Aluminum as a Risk Factor for Alzheimer's Disease," *Revista latinoamericana de enfermagem* 16, no. 1 (2008): 151–157.

11. Richard Quan, Christine Yang, Steven Rubinstein, et al., "Effects of Microwave Radiation on Anti-infective Factors in Human Milk," *Pediatrics* 89, no. 4 (April 1992): 667–669. pediatrics.aappublications.org/content/89/4/667 .abstract.

Day 6: Clean Up Your Body

1. U.S. Food and Drug Administration, "Mercury Poisoning Linked to Skin Products," last updated August 22, 2013. fda.gov/%20ForConsumers/ ConsumerUpdates/ucm294849.htm.

2. Ibid.

3. Organization for the Prohibition of Chemical Weapons, "Chemical Weapons Convention: Schedule 3." opcw.org/chemical-weapons-convention/ annex-on-chemicals/b-schedules-of-chemicals/schedule-3.

Day 7: Clean Up Your Stress

1. Mental Health America, "Americans Reveal Top Stressors, How They Cope," 2006. mentalhealthamerica.net/index.cfm?objectid=ABD3DC4E -1372-4D20-C8274399C9476E26.

2. Susan Adams, "New Survey: Majority of Employees Dissatisfied," *Forbes*, June 18, 2012.

3. Mercer Consulting Group, "One in Two US Employees Looking to Leave or Checked Out on the Job, Says *What's Working* Research," June 20, 2011. mercer.com/press-releases/1418665.

INDEX

....

Page numbers in **bold** indicate tables; those in *italics* indicate figures.